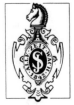

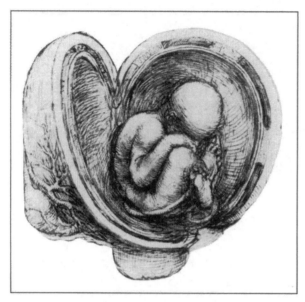

Frontispiece. Leonardo da Vinci's drawing of an embryo in utero (a detail). By gracious permission of Her Majesty The Queen.

N.B. This is one of the earliest illustrations of breech malposition, the foetal posture responsible for pre-natal hip displacement. It is a very accurate record of the left sacro-anterior lie, from the posterior aspect, being the commonest breech position; both hips are flexed and laterally rotated (see Fig. 4.13, p. 55).

John A. Wilkinson

Congenital Displacement of the Hip Joint

With 168 figures

Springer-Verlag
Berlin Heidelberg New York Tokyo

John A. Wilkinson, BSc, MCh, FRCS.

Hunterian Professor, RCS.; Simpson Smith Prize; Robert Jones Gold Medal and ABC Fellow, BOA; Senior Consultant Orthopaedic Surgeon and Clinical Teacher Southampton University Hospitals, The Lord Mayor Treloar Orthopaedic Hospital, Alton, and the Channel Islands

ISBN-13:978-1-4471-1371-3   e-ISBN-13:978-1-4471-1369-0
DOI: 10.1007/978-1-4471-1369-0

Library of Congress Cataloging in Publication Data
Wilkinson, John Arthur, 1925–   Congenital displacement of the hip joint.
Includes bibliographies and index.   1. Hip joint—Dislocation, Congenital.   I. Title.
[DNLM: 1. Hip Dislocation, Congenital. WE 860 W686c] RD772.W55 1985 617′.376 85-2584
ISBN-13:978-1-4471-1371-3 (U.S.)

© Springer-Verlag Berlin Heidelberg 1985
Softcover reprint of the hardcover 1st edition 1985

The use of registered names, trademarks etc. in this publication does not imply, even in the absence of a specific statement, that such names are exempt from the relevant laws and regulations and therefore free for general use.

Product Liability: The publisher can give no guarantee for information about drug dosage and application thereof contained in this book. In every individual case the respective user must check its accuracy by consulting other pharmaceutical literature.

2128/3916 543210

Acknowledgements

> The preparation of a monograph involves the labours, co-operation and encouragement of many individuals.
>
> *Vernon Hart* (1948)

It is my pleasure and privilege to acknowledge the efforts of many who have consciously and unconsciously contributed to the contents of this book. I am indebted to my two secretaries, Eileen Sizer and Christine Clearkin, who have worked so hard on the script, never complaining about their arduous tasks. The diagrams and photographs have been produced by the Department of Illustration, Southampton University Hospital, and I am more than grateful to Mr. David Whitcher for his advice and help, and to Mr. Peter Jack for his artistic impressions. Mrs. Janice Mayhew, the Librarian of the Wessex Regional Orthopaedic Library, has provided many of the references included in the text.

I am also indebted to the parents who have entrusted me with the care of their children, and to the nurses, physiotherapists and radiographers who have contributed to the clinical work, which has been performed at the Southampton University Hospital and the Lord Mayor Treloar Orthopaedic Hospital, Alton. I thank my colleagues who have referred their cases, and the success of my surgery has been entirely dependent upon Dr. Peter Baxter, my Senior Anaesthetist, for without his skill nothing could have been achieved.

Finally, I must address the words of John Hunter (1786) to my mentors Mr. A.O. Parker, Mr. David Trevor, Sir Herbert Seddon, Sir Denis Browne, Mr. Eric Lloyd, and Mr. George Lloyd-Roberts:

> As the following observations were made in the course of those pursuits in which you have so warmly interested yourselves and promoted with the most friendly assistance, I should be wanting in gratitude were I not to address them to you as a public testimony of the friendship and esteem with which I am, dear sirs, you obliged and very humble servant.

Southampton, January 1985   John A. Wilkinson

Preface

If I have seen further, it is by standing on ye shoulders of giants.

Sir Isaac Newton (1675)

Although congenital displacement of the hip has always been recognised as the commonest pre-natal deformity of the musculoskeletal system found in otherwise normal children, it is surprising to find that much of our present-day understanding concerning its origin and nature has been discovered only in the past 150 years and its successful management eventually emerged during the last 60 years, almost within the professional life time of our more senior colleagues.

Whereas Hippocrates (460–370 B.C.) appeared to recognise patients that had experienced dislocation of their hips in utero and identified them from acquired forms of displacement, according to Severin (1941) it was another 2000 years before Palleta (1820) first recorded a careful description of the deformity based on his observations at an autopsy performed on an 11-day-old boy with bilateral dislocations; he concluded that the findings were not caused by injury at birth, but dated from a pre-natal stage. Soon after, Baron Dupuytren (1847) gave an accurate description of congenital dislocation in his contribution entitled "Mémoire sur un déplacement original ou congénital de la tête des fémurs". He noted the absence of abscesses and fistulae as seen in painful and cruel pathological dislocations, which led him to believe that these congenital displacements were not likely to be the result of foetal disease as the affected babies appeared quite healthy at birth. He concluded that they were probably due to an accidental displacement in utero which appeared to affect girls much more frequently than boys. With amazing foresight, Dupuytren came to the conclusion that these displacements were the result of the thighs being very much bent on the belly, from which it followed that the heads of the thigh bones were continuously pressing against the lower and back part of the capsular ligaments, "a circumstance which though without effect in well-formed individuals might, I apprehend, have an injurious influence in such as are weak or of lax resisting fibre". It is no wonder that Lorenz paid tribute to Dupuytren for setting a scientific landslide in motion (Severin 1941). Yet, knowledge concerning the prevalence of this congenital deformity remained fragmentary until Roentgen (1895) discovered the diagnostic value of radiology, and soon after Le Damany and Saigret (1910) published the first detailed study in a normal population.

With regard to treatment, Pravaz (1837) was the first person known for certain to have succeeded in reducing a congenital dislocation of the hip, but again according to Severin he was unable to retain the femoral head in its new position. Poggi (1888) is thought to be the first person to have performed a successful surgical reduction, retaining the femoral head by deepening the acetabulum. His techniques were later developed by Lorenz (1896), who undertook a thorough study of the surgical anatomy of the deformation; this led him to develop his closed reduction of congenital dislocations which was referred to as the "bloodless method" by Ludloff (1913). Lorenz was the first to realise that retention of reduction by splinting was just as important as the technique of manipulative reduction. At the same time, Paci described a method of closed reduction by circumduction of the hip, and this appeared to become the more popular method in parts of Europe and England. Whereas many children under 3 years were prevented by such conservative measures from being crippled, the majority of these patients reached hospital after this age and did not respond to this treatment. Their high prevalence of redislocations and stiff hips stimulated a popular return to surgical reduction in the earlier part of this century. Major contributions were made by Hoffa (1895) and Ludloff (1913) in Europe, with Hey Groves (1928) and Fairbank (1930) in Great Britain; whereas in North America, Sherman (1903), Hibbs (1915) and Galloway (1920) were also pioneers of similar techniques. Nathaniel Allison (1928) recorded a detailed account of the history of management in his historical contribution to the Robert Jones Birthday Volume.

Later it became acknowledged generally that the results of both conservative and surgical management could only be improved upon if more cases were treated earlier, and every effort was made to bring this about. Putti (1933) produced another scientific landslide, with his concept of early diagnosis within the first year of life. He described the radiological state of "predislocation" and sincerely believed that every new-born should be subjected to a routine radiological examination. He recommended that treatment should begin at the very moment the deformity is first observed, even if it be on the day of birth, and promised a 95% cure by simply applying his adjustable abduction apparatus.

Marino Ortolani (1948) was Putti's pupil and he took a major step forward in management, by identifying hip instability clinically in the new-born. Although he gave credence to the work of his mentor, Ortolani found that the "scatto" or snapping sign was a more accurate way of diagnosing "predislocation", as compared to radiographs or even arthrography in the first year of life, and this saved exposing many normal children to radiological surveys. He found that there were "embryonary" or complete degrees of dislocation at birth which proved resistant to simple treatment. Such forms were rare compared to the commoner forms of "predislocation" or "preluxation" which were thought to develop into postnatal dislocations, although he recognised that many recovered spontaneously without treatment. Palmen (1961) carried Ortolani's methods to Scandinavia and popularised the vetting of new-born babies for hip instability throughout Sweden. Von Rosen (1962) continued with this work, enthusiastically, and Barlow brought his teaching to Great Britain. They all believed that congenital dislocation of the hip was simply a case of hip instability at the time of birth, and could be treated successfully when splinted within the first 3 days of life. Thus Andren (1961) stated "it is clear that there is hardly any excuse for congenital dislocation of the hip not being recognised and not being effectively treated from birth".

Against this background of development and modern thinking, I have gained a personal experience in the understanding of the diagnosis and treatment of this condition over the past 25 years and my findings are expounded in this monograph. As a young House Surgeon and Registrar in orthopaedic centres of excellence including the Prince of Wales Orthopaedic Hospital, the Royal National Orthopaedic Hospital, and the Hospital for Sick Children in London, I was encouraged by my mentors to discard "cant and dogma", and they stimulated me to think about the fundamental problems involved in the aetiology and management of this congenital deformity, in preference to teaching me their methods and techniques. I was directed to perform laboratory research in order to gain an understanding of the mechanism and the degrees of deformation of the normal hip joint, in immature animals exposed to the aetiological factors of hormonal joint laxity and breech malposition. The soft tissue and bony changes produced in these animals led to a basic understanding of the anatomical changes found in the hip joints of stillborn human foetuses. Thus with an intimate knowledge of the mechanism of intra-uterine hip displacement and the features and degrees of deformation, one was able to diagnose the different degrees of deformity at birth and understand the development of further changes during the first few years of life.

At that time the Ministry of Health initiated the national screening programme (1969), emphasising that "early diagnosis is therefore of greatest importance and in the earliest phases all that is required is to replace the head of the femur in the acetabulum, holding it there until the capsule shrinks and a satisfactory acetabulum forms". Such advice was not found to be fruitful and within a short time the difficulties of early diagnosis and management became apparent (Wilkinson 1972). In spite of a major effort to detect and treat affected new-born in a captive population, the prevalence of persistent hip displacement in the infant population was not reduced. Thus an original programme of treatment was evolved during my subsequent clinical experience in the Southampton University Hospitals and the Lord Mayor Treloar Orthopaedic Hospital, Alton.

Congenital displacement of the hip has been found to be partly the result of genetic and familial attributes combined with hormonal and mechanical intra-uterine factors affecting the near-normally developed foetal hip joint during the last months of pregnancy. The complexity and the degrees of deformation are not consistent, and, because of this, rigid orthodox management is doomed to failure in a large percentage of cases. It has become recognised that the primary deformation is a posterior displacement of the acetabulum affecting its three components, and a retroversion of the femur. This is associated with a recurrent displacement of the femoral head, in relation to the acetabulum, producing soft tissue deformation of the capsule and intra-articular structures.

"The term congenital dislocation of the hip which is deeply rooted in the literature does not accurately and comprehensively describe this deformity" (Gill 1948). It might be wiser to choose the term "congenital deformation of the hip" as suggested by Dunn (1976) to be a more accurate description, but this would also embrace such unrelated conditions as congenital coxa vara and other degrees of embryological failure. Therefore, I have chosen to use the terminology, "congenital displacement of the hip joint," which was first coined by Sayre (1882) and has subsequently found popularity with many writers, including Beckett Howorth (1963), and more recently Edgar Somerville (1982). Its use highlights the primary displacement of the acetabulum on the pelvis, as well as the recurrent displacement of the femoral head and the secondary soft tissue deformation.

It is hoped that the chapters of the monograph will dispel the common belief that all congenital displacements of the hip are responsive to simple treatment at birth, and also prove that the incarcerated limbus is the frequent cause of persistent displacement and iatrogenic deformation. May the evidence supplied reveal the necessity for concentric reduction, attained through excision of the limbus and maintained by the efficiency of the Lorenz splint. Finally the results of treatment will illuminate the potentials of pelvic re-orientation and decompression, compared to the morbidity of femoral realignment, in the surgical attempts to overcome incongruity of the bony components of the deformation.

"Where shall I begin, please your Majesty!" he asked. "Begin at the beginning", the King said gravely, "and go on till you come to the end: then stop".

From *Alice's Adventures in Wonderland*
by Lewis Carroll (1832–1898)

References

Andren L (1961) Aetiology and diagnosis of congenital dislocation of the hip in newborns. Radiologie (Berlin) 1:89–94

Allison N (1928) The open operations for congenital dislocation of the hip. Robert Jones Birthday Volume, Oxford University Press, Oxford

Central Health Services Council (1969) Screening for the Detection of C.D.H. in Infants. Her Majesty's Stationery Office, London

Dupuytren G (1847) Injuries and diseases of bones. Translated for the Sydenham Society, London

Dunn P (1976) Perinatal observations on the aetiology of congenital dislocation of the hip. Clinical Orthopaedics 119:11–21

Fairbank T (1930) Congenital dislocation of the hip with special reference to anatomy. Br J Surg 17:380

Galloway HPH (1920) The open operation for congenital dislocation of the hip. J Orthop Surg 2(39c)

Gill B (1948) Congenital dislocation of the hip. J Bone Joint Surg Editorial

Hart VL (1948) Congenital dysplasia of the hip joint and sequelae. Charles E. Thomas, Illinois

Hey Groves E (1928) The treatment of congenital dislocation of the hip. Robert Jones Birthday Volume, Oxford Press

Hibbs RA (1915) quoted by Nathanial Allison (1928) The open operations for congenital dislocation of the hip. Robert Jones Birthday Volume, Oxford University Press, Oxford

Hippocrates The genuine works of Hippocrates. Translation from the Greek by Francis Adams, London (1849)

Hoffa A (1895) quoted by Nathanial Allison (1928) The open operations for congenital dislocation of the hip. Robert Jones Birthday Volume, Oxford University Press, Oxford

Howorth B (1963) The etiology of congenital dislocation of the hip. Clin Orthop 29:164

Hunter J (1786) Letter to Sir Joseph Banks, President of the Royal Society

Le Damany P, Saiget J (1910) quoted by J.W. Dickson (1969) Pierre Le Damany on congenital dysplasia of the hip. Proc R Soc Med 62:575

Lorenz A (1896) Zur Priorität der unblutigen Reposition der angeborenen Hüftverrenkung. Wien klin Wchschr 9:658

Ludloff K (1913) The open reduction of the congenital hip dislocation by an anterior incision. Am J Orthop Surg 10:438–454

Newton I (1675) Newton to Hook. The correspondence of Isaac Newton, vol 1 (1661–1675). Edited by HW Turnbull, FRS

Ortolani M (1948) La lussazione congenita dell'anca: Nuovi criteri diagnostici e profillattico-correttivi. Bologna, Cappelli

Palmen K (1961) Preluxation of the hip joint. Acta Paediatr 50, Suppl 129

Poggi A (1888) Contributo alla cura cruenta della lussatione congenita. Arch Ortop p. 105

Pravaz CA (1837) Du traitment de la luxation congénitale. Bull Acad Med 2:579

Putti V (1933) Early treatment of congenital dislocation of the hip. J Bone Joint Surg 15:16

Roentgen WC (1895) Ueber eine neue Art von Strahlen (Vorlaeufige Mitteilung). Sitzungs-Berichte der Physikalisch-medizinischen Gesellschaft zu Würzburg 9:132–141

Sayre LA (1882) Orthopaedic surgery and diseases of the joints. Appleton-Century, New York

Severin E (1941) Contribution to the knowledge of congenital dislocation of the hip joint. Late results of closed reduction and arthrographic studies of recent cases. Acta Chir Scand 84, Suppl 63

Sherman H (1903) quoted by Nathanial Allison (1928) The open operations for congenital dislocation of the hip. Robert Jones Birthday Volume, Oxford University Press, Oxford

Somerville EW (1982) Displacement of the hip in childhood. Springer-Verlag, Berlin, Heidelberg, New York

Von Rosen S (1962) Diagnosis and treatment of congenital dislocation of the hip joint in the newborn. J Bone Joint Surg 44B:284

Wilkinson JA (1972) A post-natal survey for congenital displacement of the hip. J Bone Joint Surg 52B:4–49

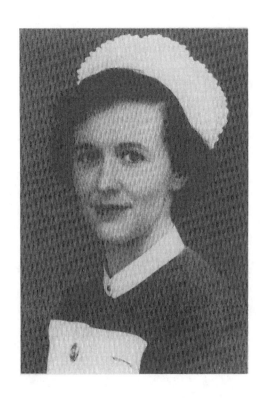

I wish to dedicate this book to
Sister Betty Paulina Keeley, S.R.N., O.N.C.,
Royal National Orthopaedic Hospital
1948–1955

Contents

1   Aetiology

Congenital dislocation of the hip joint is a deformity which is mysterious in its origin, insidious in its course and relentless in its final crippling results.

Ernest Hey Groves (1928)

By definition a congenital deformity is present at birth, being the result of interference in either early embryological development or late foetal growth in utero. When normal development is disrupted within the first 10 weeks of intra-uterine life, embryological or teratological deformities result, and the earlier the arrest, the greater the degree of malformation. Deformities resulting from early disruption of normal development are usually overt and easily diagnosed, but the early onset also lowers the potential for future development, and the response to treatment is correspondingly poor. In contrast, late interference in foetal growth produces deformities that are often difficult to diagnose and remain cryptic. Such cases have had a near-normal structural development and therefore their potential for recovery is greater, providing a better response to treatment. This explains the paradox that the more easily diagnosed congenital deformities have a poor response to treatment, whereas those that are difficult to diagnose have a greater potential for recovery.

Congenital displacement of the hip joint (CDH) has a mixed aetiology. When the developmental factors are more dominant, the displacement occurs earlier (embryological or teratological displacements), the deformity becomes more obvious by birth, but the greater degree of malformation makes spontaneous recovery less likely and the response to treatment is poor. Yet when the environmental intra-uterine factors are dominant, the displacement occurs later in pregnancy; then the diagnosis becomes more difficult, but as already pointed out, the response to treatment is better. Unfortunately,

an intermediate group of cases appears to be responsible for the increasing prevalence of persistent hip displacement in the infant population, because the diagnosis appears to be more difficult yet the response to conservative treatment is poor.

If we are to overcome the inherent problems of diagnosis and management, it is necessary for us to appreciate the degrees of variation from normal anatomy. Such knowledge can be acquired only by studying the normal human development, including the organogenesis and subsequent intra-uterine growth of the foetal limbs.

Normal Development

The duration of human intra-uterine development can be divided conveniently into four phases (Llewellyn-Jones 1972), as seen in Table 1.1. The first 10 weeks are occupied by the structural development of the embryo. Between the 10th and the 20th weeks there is an initiation and development of foetal function, while the 20th to the 40th week is occupied by the maturation of the foetus in preparation for birth and subsequent independence.

Organogenesis (Weeks 1–10)

The structural development of the embryo occupies the initial period following conception, the embryological age usually being expressed in ovulation

Table 1.1. The four quarters of pregnancy conveniently divide up intra-uterine development for practical and theoretical reasons (Llewellyn-Jones 1972)

Gestation	Stages	General features	Musculoskeletal development
Conception	1st quarter	Cephalocaudal Embryological Organogenesis	2 weeks—Limb buds appear 8 weeks—Limb buds differentiate Hip joint cleavage
10th week		Hegar's sign disappears	
	2nd quarter	Foetal development Movements—Swallowing Respiratory	Hip joint surface smooth Foetal movements—Head Arms Trunk Legs
20th week		Foetal weight 500 g Viability possible	
	3rd quarter	Mid-foetal function Radiologically apparent Ultrasonics After 28 weeks—stillborn	Universal breech posture Leg folding mechanism Total flexion posture Cephalic version
30th week		Foetal weight 1500 g Viability probable	
	4th quarter	Late foetal growth	Intra-uterine posture and presentation stabilised. Persistent lateral rotation causes hip displacement
40th week		Mean birth weight = 3500 g	
	Birth	Baby viable	Birth posture reflects previous intra-uterine final posture

weeks. The intimate details have been studied extensively in aborted specimens and the results of this research widely reported (Strayer 1943; Rooker 1979). Figure 1.1 illustrates the extent of structural development at the end of this period.

The lower limb buds appear in the 2nd week and become well differentiated by the end of the 8th week, by which time the diaphyseal ossific centres have appeared in the femur and tibia. By the 8th week the femoral and acetabular components of the embryological hip joint are separated by a cleavage, but the hip joint surfaces do not appear smooth until the 10th week and it is only then that movement can occur (personal communication from Professor Hans K. Uhthoff, Ottawa 1984).

Clinical, pathological, and experimental evidence supports the hypothesis that active movement of the embryo is required to assure normal development of the joints (Drachman and Coulombre 1962). Trueta (1968) previously suggested that this coincided with, if it were not produced by, the functional development of power in the surrounding muscles, but this theory has been challenged by

Gardener (1956). Figure 1.2 reveals joint cleavage at the 10th week.

In most synovial joints the surrounding vascular mesenchyme becomes continuous with the development of an intermediate loose layer which eventually gives rise to the capsule, synovial membrane, and intra-articular ligaments. The retro-acetabular recess appears at the 12th week, separating the capsule from the labrum. It is interesting to note that these structures arise from the same tissue and their histological appearance is identical up to the time of birth, as seen in Fig. 1.2b. This explains the difficulty experienced in identifying the origin of the limbus excised surgically after the first year.

During the embryological stage there is a general development of most systems in a cephalocaudal direction. In the central and peripheral nervous systems, this progress of development is well defined, and "all those properties which enable it to perform its regular functions are developed prior to and in the absence of all functions" (Weiss 1939). Romanes (1941) demonstrated the existence of spinal centres as anatomical entities in the human

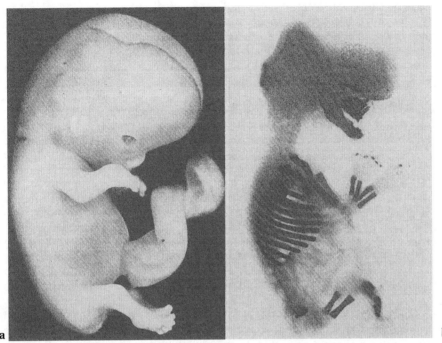

Fig. 1.1a,b. Embryo near the end of structural development (10th week) becomes lifelike and foetal; movements begin to develop. **b** reveals the ossific centres present at the end of the 10th week. (Fig. 1.1b from Brookes 1973, with permission)

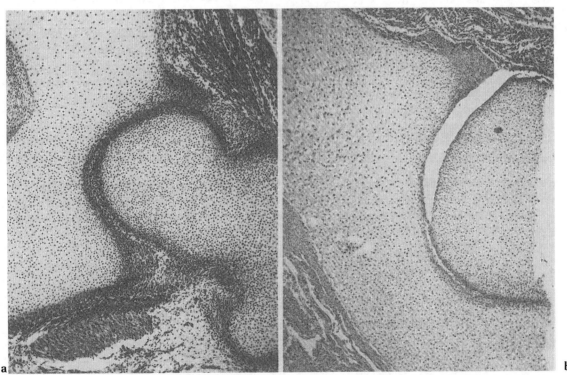

Fig. 1.2a,b. Development of joint cleavage. **a** Hip joint cavity appearing at 8th week. **b** Labrum separating from hip capsule at 12th week, each arising from the same mesenchyme and having the same structural appearance. (By courtesy of Professor Hans Uhthoff, University of Ottawa)

foetus, and Last (1949) suggested that these were spinal segmental centres for joint movements. The progressive anatomical innervation of the lower limbs involves the successive segmental distribution of the lumbosacral plexus from the lower thoracic to the upper sacral levels.

Thus, at the end of the 10th week structural development is almost complete, the embryo is life-like in appearance and functional development begins. It is at this stage that it is called a foetus.

Early Foetal Development (Weeks 10–20)

Unlike the previous embryological phase, early foetal development remains cryptic, as the human foetal function cannot be observed directly for ethical reasons. Foetal ages are usually measured in menstrual weeks and to understand the development of function and the growth changes in the earlier stages, one is dependent upon animal studies and conjecture. Stimulation of cat foetuses at successive stages of development indicates that there is an increasing wealth of muscular contractions appearing in the same cephalocaudal direction as the preceding embryological development. In the hind limb, active hip flexion is followed by knee extension and later knee flexion, while the foot movements appear subsequently (Weiss 1939). If this thesis is accepted, the theoretical appearance of muscle function and dominance resulting in move-

ments and posture is dependent upon the levels of innervation in the spinal cord. The first muscle to be innervated is the psoas (lumbar 1, 2, and 3) which flexes and adducts the thigh (McKibbin 1968). Later the quadriceps, innervated by lumbar 2, 3, and 4, extends the knee joint, as seen in Fig. 1.3.

As early foetal posture is the result of sustained muscular contractions acting upon the individual joints, the foetus must first assume hip flexion and adduction associated with knee extension. A further spread of sustained contractions to the other muscle groups motivates the folding mechanism of the foetal legs, the iliopsoas and hip adductors rotating the thigh laterally with the help of the lateral rotators (lumbar 2, 3, and 4), and this is followed by dorsiflexion of the foot before knee flexion. Generally dorsal innervation precedes ventral, and this means at the L4, L5, and S1 levels, dorsiflexion of the foot occurs before knee flexion, the latter being due to the development of power in the medial hamstrings. Bobath (1966) observed the same cephalocaudal spread of autonomic reactions for the maintenance of posture and equilibrium in normal babies, postnatally, during the first 10 months of life.

Mid-Foetal Development (Weeks 20–30)

During this second half of pregnancy foetal movements and posture can be studied in the human by

DEVELOPMENTAL INNERVATION of the LEGS		
	ANATOMICAL	**POSTURAL**
Lumbar 1	Psoas	
2	Quadriceps	Extended knee posture
3		
4	Lateral Rotators	
Lumbar 5	Hamstrings	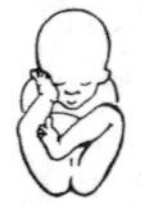 Lateral rotational leg – folding mechanism
Sacral 1	Foot Dorsiflexors	
Sacral 1	Gluteus Medius	Medial rotation of flexed thighs
2	Gluteus Maximus	

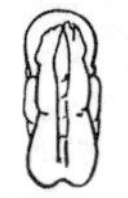

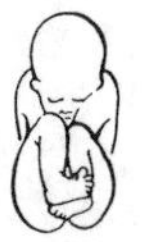

Fig. 1.3. Theoretical development of anatomical innervation and subsequent muscle function, with acquired foetal postures. (Wilkinson 1980, with permission)

ultrasonic and radiological surveys, but unfortunately the risk of exposure to the foetus limits such examinations and restricts the source of information. Vartan (1945) performed an extensive radiological survey on 4000 pregnancies, before such risks were appreciated, and he discovered that breech presentation was so common before the 28th week that it could be considered normal at this stage. When the knees were hyperextended and uncrossed, the legs frequently failed to fold and the foetus remained locked in the extended breech malposition, as seen in Fig. 1.4. This prevented spontaneous cephalic version and the pregnancies terminated in breech deliveries.

In the majority of breech presentations the foetal legs were semi-flexed and crossed and these underwent spontaneous version before the 30th week, being delivered normally (see Fig. 1.5).

We are fortunate to have this research, even with its limitations, as it supports the theoretical patterns of postural development already described. Russell (1969) reviewed the radiographs of 145 singleton

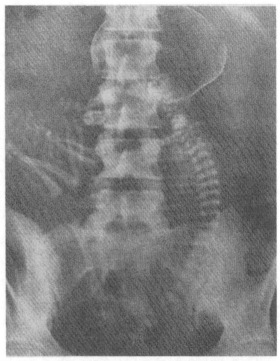

Fig. 1.5. Radiological appearance of foetal posture before the 30th week—semi-flexed breech. Note the breech presentation: the knees are semi-flexed and the lower legs crossed. (Wilkinson 1966, with permission)

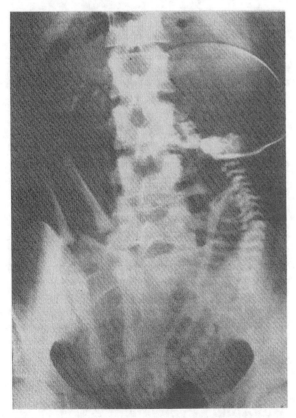

Fig. 1.4. Radiological appearance of foetal posture before the 30th week—hyperextended breech. Note the breech presentation: the knees are extended and the lower legs uncrossed. The foetal head and spine are on the same side of the maternal spine. (Wilkinson 1966, with permission)

breech pregnancies and confirmed the "rule of the side of the head": if the foetal head lies on the same side of the mother as the foetal spine, the legs are usually extended (see Fig. 1.4). If the head is on the opposite side of the maternal spine to the foetal spine, the legs are usually flexed. This rule appeared to be positive in nearly 80% of cases and confirmed that it is necessary for the foetal hips and knees to flex before spinal flexion and version can take place, as shown in Fig. 1.6.

Normally the foetus passes through the successive stages of leg-folding, reaching the final stage of intra-uterine posture before the 28th week. The legs are then flexed at the hips and knees and this allows spinal and cephalic flexion. The foetus becomes wrapped in a ball, in its most stable posture, the hips and thighs being flexed and medially rotated. The knees are also flexed and the foot is held in calcaneus. The universal tendency for cephalic presentation still remains one of the greatest mysteries of intra-uterine development. Spontaneous version usually occurs before the 30th week and the commonest cause preventing it taking place is the persistent extension of the foetal knees, as this interferes with the required degree of spinal flexion. Beyond

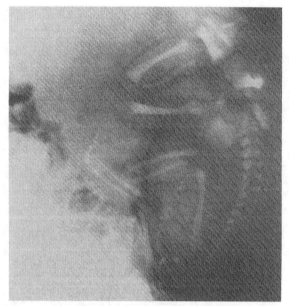

Fig. 1.6. Radiological appearance of foetal posture after the 32nd week—full flexion. Note the cephalic presentation: the knees, hips and spine are fully flexed.

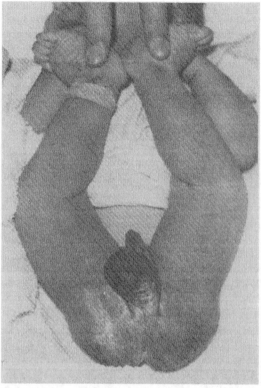

Fig. 1.7 Birth posture—breech presentation. Note the caput, involving the buttocks, and the semi-flexed knees laterally rotated—the lateral rotation breech position. (Wilkinson 1963, with permission)

the 28th week such posture is abnormal and constitutes malposition. The latter is more common in primiparous pregnancies, owing to the natural oligohydramnios which restricts foetal movements and interferes with the leg-folding mechanism. Thus there is a higher prevalence of breech malposition and breech presentation in first-born babies. Amniocentesis is also reported to have a similar effect.

Late Foetal Development (Weeks 30–40)

Birth postures are an accurate record of the pre-existing pre-natal posture in which the foetus has been wrapped up during the last 8 weeks or more of pregnancy. Normally the posture persists for a few days and then gradually disappears, as the newborn adapts to its new-found freedom. Chapple and Davidson (1941) stressed the value of recording these postures before they were lost, "so that certain obscure deformities not apparent on ordinary inspection might be detected", as seen in Fig. 1.7.

Before the 28th week of pregnancy there is usually enough liquor for the foetus to move its limbs freely. This allows frequent changes of posture, the limbs tending to return to the position dictated by the dominant muscle groups. After the 28th week the rapid growth of the foetus obliterates much of the intra-uterine space, and the longer legs become more confined to their planes of movement than the

shorter arms. The legs are usually restricted to the plane of rotation, either medially or laterally. Thus birth moulding records the features of this final posture and they are more marked in the fully mature foetus. Obviously there is less evidence of sustained intra-uterine posture in premature births, except in primiparous pregnancies, where there is a natural oligohydramnios. Post-natal surveys have revealed evidence of minimal delay in leg-folding in normal cephalic deliveries, as compared with maximal delay in the leg-folding mechanism of breech births (Wilkinson 1972; see Fig. 5.3). This reflects the importance of a physiological arrest in leg-folding in otherwise normal pregnancies, producing premature births because the unfolded foetus occupies too much intra-uterine space.

Abnormal Development

As soon as it became recognised that intra-uterine development could be arrested at varying stages, resulting in abnormal growth patterns, a number of theories were propounded as to the exact nature of such interference and the timing of their influence on the growth of the embryo and foetus. Such aetiological theories of congenital deformation became divided into two conflicting schools: the developmental and the environmental. The former embraced a number of embryological theories, whereas the latter was based on mechanical and also hormonal disturbances in the intra-uterine foetal development.

Embryological Theories

Sir Arthur Keith (1948) expressed the developmental theory, as he believed that congenital deformities were malformations resulting from an interference with the normal stages of embryological development. Sex-linked genes were first held to be responsible, but the experiments of Duraiswami (1952) focused attention on previous work performed on toxic teratological agents, which affected the developing organism to produce multiple abnormalities in various systems, according to the stage of organogenesis in which they are introduced. Duraiswami injected insulin, which interfered with the carbohydrate metabolism of the embryological nervous system.

In 1949 a new concept originated in the developmental school when Badgeley revived the work of Le Damany (1914), who believed femoral anteversion to be the most important anatomical feature producing intra-uterine hip displacement. Badgeley applied the principles of dynamic development propounded by Weiss (1939) and formed the opinion that the primary cause was a partial failure of the leg to rotate medially, before the joint space had appeared between the cartilaginous components of the hip. This interfered with local growth adjustments and resulted in femoral anteversion combined with anterior acetabular dysplasia. These reciprocal deformities were finally responsible for producing anterior displacement of the hip joint in utero.

Hormonal Theories

Softening and lengthening of the maternal pelvic ligaments during pregnancy produces a pliancy of the birth canal that facilitates labour. Hisaw (1926) was able to induce these changes under endocrine control in both immature and mature female guinea-pigs by injecting them with oestrone followed by progesterone. No such laxity appeared in immature male animals. He later isolated relaxin to be the responsible hormone produced by the oestrogen-sensitised uterus as a normal response to progesterone (Hisaw et al. 1944). Aqueous luteal extracts containing relaxin were discovered by Martin and Schoenbach (1959) and they proved that the hormone was a protein of low molecular weight. It was found in the maternal blood serum of rabbits, guinea-pigs, sows, and women and the hormonal effects were demonstrated on the pubic symphyses and sacro-iliac joints of guinea-pigs and rabbits. Hormonal joint laxity was not confined to pregnant animals, as immature females developed similar changes in response to oestrone and progesterone injections, but male animals and hysterectomised females were unaffected. The same degree of laxity was demonstrated in the hips and knees of immature rabbits (Wilkinson 1963). Experimental studies on the effects of the sex hormones on the elastic fibre of capsular ligaments in the hip joint were performed in Kyoto University by Yamamuro et al. in 1977. Their results suggested that oestrogen inhibited collagen synthesis and accelerated collagen cross-linkage and elastin formation in the hip joint capsule, while progesterone and testosterone had the opposite effect. Thus connective tissue formation in the hip joint capsule appeared to be controlled by the hormonal environment. These animal experiments led the authors to believe that oestrogen inhibited the development of hip displacement, while progesterone tended to promote it.

With regard to human foetal endocrinology, problems exist because the foetus is too old for the embryologist and too young for the endocrinologist, and this has led to its neglect (Jost 1953). The hormonal *milieu intérieur* of the human foetus is dependent upon the balance between the supply and metabolism of maternal placental and foetal sources. Another controlling factor is the placento-amniotic barrier between the maternal and foetal circulations. This prevents many of the maternal hormones, especially proteins, from reaching the foetus. The passage of foetal hormones into the maternal circulation is less restricted and many are metabolised and excreted. Placental hormones have a free access to the foetal circulation because they are produced in the foetal trophoblast (Jost 1953). In the first trimester the maternal ovaries are the only source of oestrogens and progesterone, but the chorion prevents them and relaxin from entering the foetal circulation (Diczfalusy et al. 1961). During the third phase, placental oestrone and progesterone pass into the foetal circulation. The active oestrone and oestradiol-17B are conjugated normally by the foetal liver to form inactive oestriol, and similarly active progesterone is converted to inactive pregnandiol (Andren and Borglin 1961). Oestriol and pregnandiol enter the maternal circulation and are excreted. During the fourth phase the placental trophoblast degenerates and its hormonal production is discontinued, but then maternal gonadotrophins stimulate the foetal adrenal glands to produce progesterone (Forbes 1955) and the foetal ovaries secrete oestrone (Pinkerton 1959). This is probably the most important period of foetal endocrinology with regard to the aetiology of pre-natal hip displacement and it continues until birth. Thus active oestrone and progesterone are present in small amounts in the foetal serum during the second half of pregnancy. They produce hormonal joint laxity by their direct action on the foetal liga-ments and also stimulate the immature uterus to produce relaxin. This hormone has a more relaxing effect upon the female foetal ligaments. The sex dif-ference would be more apparent if the foetal blood levels of active oestrone and progesterone were not controlled by the conjugation of these active hor-mones in the foetal liver, which converts them into their inactive forms. Andren and Borglin (1961) claimed to have discovered a failure of this hepatic function in children with congenital hip displace-ment, causing an increase in the degree of foetal hormonal laxity.

Chapple and Davidson (1941) were the first to recognise the significance of Dr Pendleton Tomkins' discovery that ligamentous structures in the foetus may be relaxed by the relaxing hormone of the mother. He found it comparable to other hormonal effects, including vaginal discharge and breast enlargement, and felt it might account for the sex linkage of CDH. Such a temporary instability of the female foetal hip joints would make them more sus-ceptible to mechanical factors.

Mechanical Theories

The hypothesis that feet and limbs can be moulded by pressure and malposition before birth may be called the Hippocratic theory after its first known proponent. With regard to CDH, Lorenz (1920) was the first to point out that the majority of affected infants responded well to conservative treatment and appeared to have normally developed hip joints affected by temporary dysplasia. The degree of recovery revealed a far greater growth potential than one would expect to find in long-standing intra-uterine malformations and was more typical of a dislocation occurring probably within the last few months of pregnancy. He believed that the

mechanism of intra-uterine hip displacement was dependent upon an acute flexion posture of the foetal hip joint producing postero-inferior hip dis-placement. Clarke (1910) had previously recognised the over-flexed position of the thighs in a new-born breech presentation and felt that this was the aetio-logical mechanical factor. Browne (1936) reverted to the Hippocratic mechanical theories of intra-uterine deformation, believing that even in the presence of normal intra-uterine posture the uterine wall could produce a thrust on the flexed knee, forc-ing the head of the femur downwards and back-wards, so that when acetabular dysplasia was present displacement of the femoral head took place. More recently Yamamuro et al. (1977) suggested that persistent knee extension was a common mechanical factor in the production of hip displace-ment and noted its prevalence in association with breech malposition.

In retrospect Tubby (1912) overcame any objec-tions to such dynamic and mechanical theories by introducing a third dimension when he stated that "we are not concerned with any particular evil or abnormal position adopted in utero, as almost any position if maintained too long leads to a definite result". He believed that the intra-uterine mechan-ism of hip displacement might well depend upon a "persistence of malposition" which is temporal rather than spatial in nature. Experiments per-formed by Drachman and Coulombre (1962) pro-vided the proof of this theory, by suggesting that there may be many unknown factors responsible for a temporary paralysis or delay in the functional development of the foetal neural system. They injec-ted fertilised eggs with curare and scoline at varying stages of functional development and were able to produce congenital deformities of the legs and feet of the chicks. The postures of the deformed limbs reflected the embryonic position of the chick and were influenced by the contour of the calcareous shell. Their experimental evidence supported the hypothesis that active movement of the embryo is required to assure normal development of the joints and even a temporary interference of muscle activity can cause deformation.

The Mechanism of CDH

Much of our knowledge concerning the develop-ment of intra-uterine posture and hip displacement has been gained from foetal diseases which interfere with the normal development of innervation and muscle function in utero. These arrests of develop-

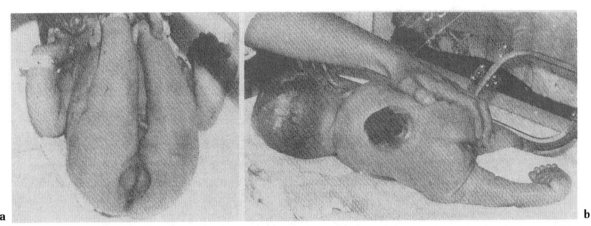

a   b

Fig. 1.8a,b. New-born babe with meningomyelocele. Breech delivery, hyperextended knees, the hamstrings never having been innervated. See birth posture.

ment cause the persistence of normal postures up to the time of birth. Sharrard (1964) plotted the innervation of the lower limb muscle groups through the lumbosacral plexus by stimulating the exposed spinal cords of new-born suffering from meningomyeloceles and found that the degrees of paralysis were congruous with the varying patterns of posture. Such postural deformities can be recognised at birth and reflect the degree of paralysis resulting from the levels of interference with the normal leg-folding mechanism. Many of these babies are breech born and have congenital displacement of their hips and knee joints (see Fig. 1.8). Similar patterns of posture are also seen in babies with arthrogryphosis. Brown et al. (1980) recorded the correlation of these patterns of deformity with the clinical paralysis in the new-born, as seen in Fig. 1.9.

Thus an anatomical or even a physiological arrest of the leg-folding mechanism of the foetus, between the 25th and 30th weeks of intra-uterine life, imposes a locked breech posture upon the foetus; this has become recognised as the "position of dislocation" (Wilkinson 1972; see Fig. 1.10). If one

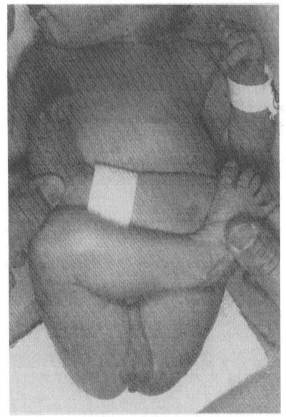

Fig. 1.10. Position of dislocation. Note that the tibia is imposing 90° of lateral torsion on the femur and flexed hip joint. Cf. Frontispiece. (Wilkinson 1972, with permission)

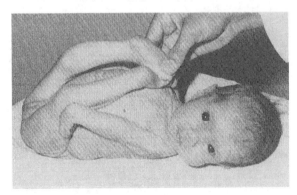

Fig. 1.9. New-born babe with arthrogryphosis. Breech delivered, the birth posture correlating with the degree of muscle paresis involving the hamstrings. (Wilkinson 1963, with permission)

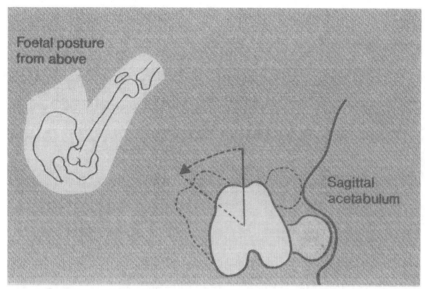

Fig. 1.11. Mechanism of hip displacement in utero, remembering that the hip remains flexed before birth, and looking from the knee above, down the shaft of the femur to the hip below. Lateral rotation of the femur can be seen to displace the head posteriorly, over the posterior rim of the acetabulum. This displacement is prevented by the development of femoral and acetabular retroversion.

views the flexed hip from above, looking from the knee to the hip below, it can be seen that lateral rotation of the femur displaces the femoral head over the posterior rim of the acetabulum, as seen in Fig. 1.11). This can only occur when there is a laxity of the capsular ligaments. Such a mechanism also produces retroversion of the femur and acetabulum, which allows the flexed hip to assume the position of lateral rotation in the absence of hip displacement, when the capsular ligaments are normal (see Chap. 2).

Summary

Thus the crux of this thesis is that a physiological delay of the normal leg-folding process in the development of foetal posture produces a persistent lateral rotation malposition on the flexed hip joint, which can result in both soft tissue and bony deformation and can lead to either temporary or persistent displacement of the human hip during its pre-natal development.

References

Andren L, Borglin NE (1961) Disturbed urinary excretion pattern of oestrogen in newborns with congenital dislocation of the hip. Acta Endocrinol 37:423–427

Badgeley CE (1949) Etiology of congenital dislocation of the hip. J Bone Joint Surg 31A:341

Bobath K (1966) Motor deficit in patients with cerebral palsy. London Spastic International Medical Publications in association with William Heinemann. Clinics in Dev. Med. No. 23

Brown LM, Robson MJ, Sharrard WJW (1980) The pathophysiology of arthrogryphosis multiplex congenita neurologica. J Bone Joint Surg 62B:291

Browne D (1936) Congenital deformities of mechanical origin. Proc R Soc Med 29:1409

Chapple CC, Davidson TD (1941) A study of the relationship between foetal position and certain congenital deformities. J Paediatrics 18:483

Clarke JJ (1910) Congenital dislocation of the hip. Ballière, Tindall & Cox, London

Diczfalusy E, Cassmer O, Alonso C, de Miquel M (1961) Oestrogen metabolism in the human foetus. Acta Endocrinol 37:353

Drachman DB, Coulombre AJ (1962) Experimental clubfoot and arthrogryphosis multiplex congenita. Lancet 523

Duraiswami PK (1952) Experimental causation of congenital skeletal defects and its significance in orthopaedic surgery. J Bone Joint Surg 34B:646–698

Forbes TR (1955) Apparent secretion of progesterone by human and goat foetuses. Endocrinology 56:699

Gardener E (1956) The development and growth of bones and joints. The American Academy of Orthopaedic Surgeons' Instructional Course of Lectures, Chap. 6

Hey Groves E (1928) The treatment of congenital dislocation of the hip joint with special reference to open operative reduction. The Robert Jones Birthday Volume. Oxford University Press, Oxford, p 73

Hisaw FL (1926) Experimental relaxation of the pubic ligaments in the guinea pig. Proc Soc Exp Biol Med 23:661

Hisaw FL, Zarrow MX, Money WL, Talmage R, Abramowitz A (1944) Importance of female reproductive tract in the formation of relaxin endocrinology. Endocrinology 34(2):122

Jost A (1953) Problems of fetal endocrinology—The gonadal and hypopophyseal hormones. Recent Prog Horm Res 8:379

Keith A (1948) Human embryology and morphology, 6th edn. Arnold, London

Last RJ (1949) Innervation of the limb. J Bone Joint Surg 31B:452

Le Damany P (1914) Congenital luxation of the hip. Am J Surg 11(4):541

Lorenz A (1920) Die sogenannte angeborene Huftverrenkung. Deutsche Orthopaedie, Stuttgart

Llewellyn-Jones D (1972) The four quarters of pregnancy. Lancet 2:737

Martin JM, Schoenbach H (1959) Historical aspects of relaxin. Ann NY Acad Sci 75:923

McKibbin B (1968) The action of the ileopsoas muscle in the newborn. J Bone Joint Surg 50B:161

Pinkerton JHM (1959) Oestrogen production in the immature human ovary. Br J Obstet Gynaecol 66(5):820

Romanes GJ (1941) Cell columns in the spinal cord of the human foetus of 14 weeks. J Anat 75:145

Rooker GD (1979) The embryological congruity of the hip joint. Ann R Coll Surg 61(5):357

Russell JGB (1969) The position of the lower limbs in breech presentations. J Obstet Gynaecol 76(4):351

Sharrard WJW (1964) Posterior iliopsoas transplantation in the treatment of paralytic dislocation of the hip. J Bone Joint Surg 46B:426

Strayer LM (1943) The embryology of the human hip joint. Yale J Biol Med 16:13–26

Trueta J (1968) Studies of the development and decay of the human frame. Heinemann, London

Tubby AH (1912) Deformities including diseases of the bones and joints. Macmillan, London

Vartan CK (1945) The behaviour of the foetus in utero with special reference to the incidence of breech presentation at term. J Obstet Gynaecol 52:417

Weiss P (1939) Principles of development. Holt, New York

Wilkinson JA (1963) Prime factors in the aetiology of congenital dislocation of the hip. J Bone Joint Surg 45B:268

Wilkinson JA (1966) Breech malposition and intra-uterine dislocations. Proc R Soc Med 59(11):1106–1108

Wilkinson JA (1972) A post-natal survey for congenital displacement of the hip. J Bone Joint Surg 54B:4

Wilkinson JA (1980) Results of surgical treatment in congenital dislocation of the hip. Isr J Med Sci 16:281–283

Yamamuro T, Hama H, Takeda T (1977) Biomechanical and hormonal factors in the etiology of congenital dislocation of the hip joint. Internat Orthop (SICOT) 1231:231

2 Experimental Research

I trust that the observations of others may, at some future period, furnish an interpretation of this phenomenon, and complete that which I have failed to establish in the history of this singular affection.

Baron Dupuytren (1847)

The effects of persistent posture on bone growth were first studied experimentally by Professor Appleton of Cambridge (1934). He then defined a postural deformity in its simplest form as:

> consisting of the persistence of an adoption of some posture which though unusual is yet within the range of postures of the normal individual. Such a persistence also leads to alteration in the soft tissues, especially involving the shortening of muscles and ligaments which set a limit to the movement and variations of posture. Subsequent changes commonly occur in the bone formation.

Appleton investigated the effects of posture by applying splints and by interfering with the nerve supply to single muscle groups. He came to the conclusion that his experiments showed that changes in the form of healthy bone resulted from the adoption of unusual postures in growing animals. Such changes did not appear after the obliteration of the epiphyseal lines and in skeletally mature animals. His experiments included the study of torsional forces acting in the plane of the epiphyses, as well as compressive forces applied at right angles. In retrospect this paper is a fundamental contribution to the understanding of the effects of breech malposition on the intra-uterine growth of the soft tissues and the bony components of the foetal hip joint, especially with regard to the torsional modifications of the femur.

Rotational Splinting

It was necessary to repeat these experiments, focusing attention on the biomechanics of the immature hip joint (Wilkinson 1962). It was found that sustained medial rotation of the hind limb in the immature rabbit, produced by the application of a plaster spica, resulted in femoral anteversion (Fig. 2.1), whereas sustained lateral rotation produced retroversion of the femur (Fig. 2.2).

A more careful examination of the rabbit's femurs indicated that most of the torsional deformity was localised in the distal femoral metaphysis, there being little deformity in the proximal third of the shaft. Initially it was felt that this was due to unequal distribution of growth, as occurs in the human femur, where two thirds of the growth occurs in the distal epiphysis (Gill and Abbott 1942). Later studies, however, showed that the metaphyseal growth in the rabbit was equally distributed between distal and proximal femoral epiphyses. It was eventually concluded that the torsional forces were transmitted by the collateral ligaments of the knee to act directly on the distal femoral epiphyses, whereas its effects had to be transmitted through the length of the diaphysis to act upon the proximal epiphyses. The latter was also protected by the iliopsoas tendon, as well as by the capsule of the hip joint, as shown in Fig. 2.3.

Thus, Appleton's findings were confirmed with regard to the rotational forces in the plane of the epiphysis producing torsional changes in the metaphyses, the rotation of the deformity being in the opposite direction to the deforming force.

Lorenz Splint Mechanism

The simple rotational experiments suggested that the Lorenz position (90° of abduction and flexion in neutral rotation) corrected femoral retroversion, and so experiments were performed to observe its effects on femoral anteversion. The outcome showed that there was a gradual correction of pre-existing anteversion in animals splinted in Lorenz plasters (Wilkinson 1962), as explained in Fig 2.4.

A study of Fig. 2.4 reveals the mechanism of the Lorenz splint. When an anteverted femur is flexed and abducted, the thigh has to be laterally rotated

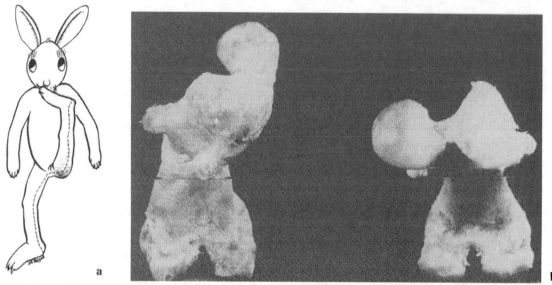

Fig. 2.1a,b. Medial rotation splinting of immature rabbit's hind leg (left). This produced excessive femoral anteversion on the splinted side in 6–12 weeks. See left femur compared to retroverted unsplinted right femur (normal). (Wilkinson 1963, with permission)

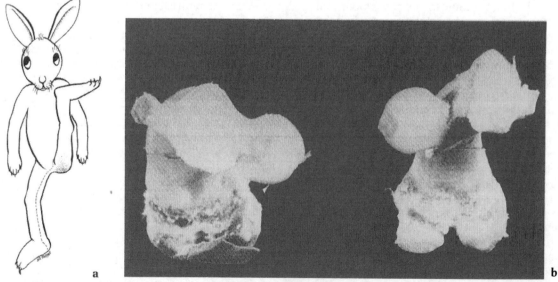

Fig. 2.2a,b. Lateral rotation splinting of immature rabbit's hind leg (left). This produced excessive femoral retroversion on the splinted side in 6–12 weeks. The left femur is more retroverted than the unsplinted right femur (normal). (Wilkinson 1963, with permission)

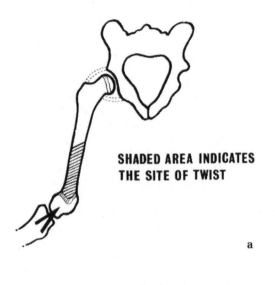

SHADED AREA INDICATES
THE SITE OF TWIST

a

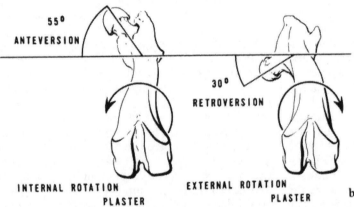

55°
ANTEVERSION

30°
RETROVERSION

INTERNAL ROTATION
PLASTER

EXTERNAL ROTATION
PLASTER   b

Fig. 2.3a,b. Mechanism and distribution of torsional deformation of the femur, in the absence of hormonal joint laxity. **a** Distribution mainly affecting the distal femoral metaphysis, the torsion being transmitted through the collateral ligaments of the knee to act directly on the distal femoral epiphysis, whereas the proximal femoral epiphysis is protected by the capsular ligament and iliopsoas muscle (Wilkinson 1963, with permission). **b** Anticlockwise, medial torsion produces femoral anteversion. Clockwise, lateral torsion produces femoral retroversion (Wilkinson 1962, with permission).

Fig. 2.4. Mechanism of the Lorenz splint in correcting excessive anteversion and retroversion. The anteverted femur has to be rotated laterally to attain the neutral position and this torsion corrects the primary deformity. Similarly the retroverted femur is rotated medially. (Wilkinson 1962, with permission)

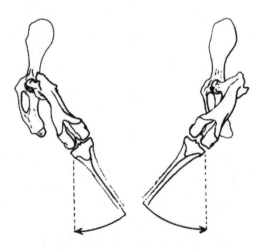

ANTEVERSION   RETROVERSION

to bring the lower leg into the same vertical plane as the trunk, and the extent of lateral rotation required is dependent upon the degree of femoral anteversion present. The lateral rotation strain placed upon the thigh corrects the anteversion. The same mechanism applies to the retroverted femur, which has to be medially rotated to bring the shin into line with the trunk. This medial rotation strain corrects the retroversion. Thus the rotational force required to bring the limb into the true Lorenz position will automatically tend to correct any preexisting femoral anteversion or retroversion.

Compression Experiments

Appleton's experiments involving compressive forces, acting at right angles to the epiphyses, were repeated by Arkin and Katz (1956), who applied angular splints to the knees of rabbits. They confirmed the original findings that lesser postural pressures slowed and retarded growth, whereas it took up to 400 lb/in.^{2} to inhibit the upper tibial epiphyseal growth in the rabbit. In addition their experiments appeared to uphold the Huerter-Volkmann law (1862; quoted by Arkin and Katz 1956), which stated that increased pressure inhibited epiphyseal growth while decreased pressure accelerated it. To investigate this, Wilkinson (1967) performed a series of experiments on the effects of compression and decompression on the growth of the epiphyses, achieved by lengthening and shortening the intervening diaphysis, as shown in Fig. 2.5.

Control experiments were undertaken dividing the diaphysis at its midpoint and using intramedull-

ary wires with an intervening metal disc at the site of osteotomy. This was to ensure that the disturbance of intramedullary blood supply did not have an adverse effect upon the proximal and distal epiphyses. Metal tags were placed in the distal epiphysis and metaphysis, on both sides of the growth plate, in order to measure accurately the distal femoral growth. Another metal tag was placed proximal to the site of the osteotomy to make sure there was no loss of diaphyseal length at this level. The proximal epiphyseal growth was measured from the overall length of the bone, subtracting the other two readings. At the time of animal sacrifice, the arterial system was outlined by injection of Micropaque in order to see whether there had been any change in the distribution of the nutrient vessels. Twelve control animals showed that there was no increase or decrease in the overall growth of the femur, at the site of osteotomy and the distal metaphysis, indicating that there was no change in the proximal epiphyseal growth, as shown in Fig. 2.6.

When the diaphysis was shortened, by removing 1 cm of the shaft at the site of osteotomy, there was no evidence of any stimulation of either the distal or the proximal epiphyseal growth. The femurs remained 1 cm short up to the time of skeletal maturity, when the animals were sacrificed.

When the diaphysis was lengthened by inserting a 1-cm-long disc at the site of osteotomy, there was a subsequent loss of leg length. In 13 successful experiments the 1-cm lengthening was reduced to almost 0.5 cm by the time skeletal maturity was attained, and much of that loss was in the proximal femoral epiphysis.

Thus these experiments proved that compression of an epiphysis, by lengthening the diaphysis, depressed proximal and distal growth; but there was no evidence to suggest that decompression, by shortening the diaphysis, accelerated juxta-epiphyseal growth.

Experiments Studying the Effects of Breech Malposition and Hormonal Joint Laxity

Unfortunately all the previous experiments were not sufficient to explain the postural changes occurring in the human femurs in utero as a result of breech malposition. The experimental findings were dependent upon forces transmitted by the capsular and collateral ligaments, but it was known that in the human foetus maternal hormones produced a

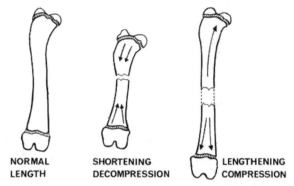

NORMAL   SHORTENING   LENGTHENING
LENGTH   DECOMPRESSION   COMPRESSION

Fig. 2.5. Experiments involving the shortening and lengthening of the diaphysis in the growing femur, to study the effects of decompressing and compressing the juxta-epiphyseal growth plates.

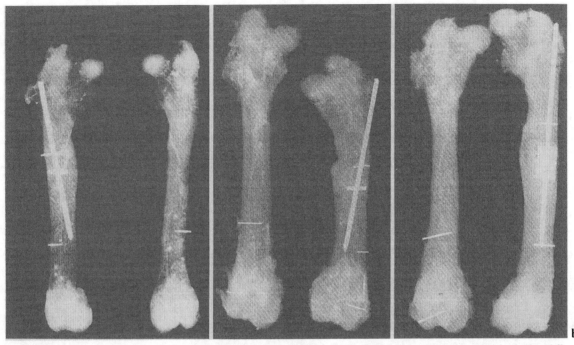

a   b,c

Fig. 2.6a–c. Results of shortening and lengthening the intervening diaphysis at 6 weeks. The animals were sacrificed when fully grown and their femurs were measured. As compared to the control group (**a**), femoral shortening persisted (**b**), but lengthening was subsequently lost (**c**) because of the compression of the juxta-epiphyses.

generalised joint laxity, especially in the female (see section on hormonal joint laxity in Chap. 1). Such generalised ligamentous laxity might disrupt any transfer of torsional forces transmitted through the capsular ligaments. It was therefore decided to repeat the series of torsional experiments on animals in which joint laxity had been produced by injecting oestrone and progesterone, before imposing a persistent malposition by splinting one of the hind limbs in flexion and either medial or lateral rotation.

The hormones had a greater effect upon the immature female rabbits than upon the males. This was thought to be due to either a greater degree of inactivation of the hormones by the male liver, or a stimulated hypertrophy of the female uterus to produce its own progesterone and add to the effect of the injected hormones. It was found that the ligamentous laxity prevented the development of femoral torsion by the interference of the transmitted forces through the relaxed collateral ligaments of the knee joint, as seen in Fig. 2.7. The femurs were found to develop anteversion or retroversion in the proximal metaphyses, but this appeared to be due to an unequal pressure on the proximal epiphysis, which hindered either anterior or posterior growth respectively. The deformities were not so grotesque or severe as those produced in the non-hormonal series. This was thought to be due to the fact that the laxity allowed the rabbit to adopt the

breech posture, without undue force being applied to the articulations of the hind limb.

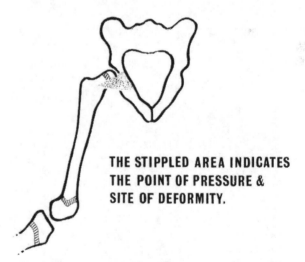

THE STIPPLED AREA INDICATES THE POINT OF PRESSURE & SITE OF DEFORMITY.

Fig. 2.7. Mechanism and distribution of femoral deformation and absence of torsional deformity in the presence of hormonal laxity. Compression of the proximal epiphysis produced cervical anteversion. (Wilkinson 1963, with permission)

Medial Rotational Splinting

When the prepared animals were splinted in medial rotational breech posture with the knees extended,

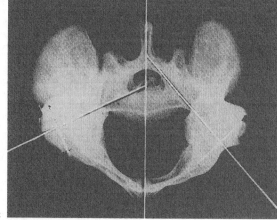

displacement did not appear to take place in the hip joint in the weekly radiographs taken during the period of splinting. After 6 weeks the animals were sacrificed and it was found that the femurs had developed proximal anteversion associated with an anteversion of the ipsilateral acetabulum, as shown in Fig. 2.8. It was seen that the distal half of the femur was not deformed. When the proximal epiphysis was sectioned, there was no evidence of any change in the thickness of the epiphyseal plate, but the height of the epiphysis anteriorly was reduced when compared with the posterior aspect of the femoral head. Similar changes have been reported subsequently in experiments imposing compression on the proximal femoral epiphyses in piglets (Graham Hall 1981). Figure 2.9 shows a diagrammatic cross-section of the femoral epiphyses.

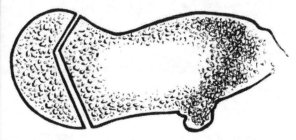

Fig. 2.9. Proximal femoral anteversion produced by compression of the anterior (upper) aspect of the epiphysis. Note the loss in anterior epiphyseal height, compared to the posterior aspect.

In some of the female rabbits, the splinted knees hyperextended and displaced, but the hips remained undisplaced radiographically (Fig. 2.10). Examination of the intra-articular structure of these hips at necropsy revealed a thinning of the articular cartilage over the posterior part and a total loss over the anterior part of the acetabulum as compared with the opposite hip. This suggested that there may have been a tendency for anterior subluxation of the femoral head during the period of splinting, as seen in Fig. 2.11.

Lateral Rotational Splinting

The response of the conditioned animals treated in lateral rotational breech posture differed according to sex. The males appeared to develop a lesser degree of hormonal laxity, and during the experiment there was no radiological evidence of hip dislocation. At the end of 6 weeks, necropsy revealed some changes in the soft tissues, especially the posterior capsule

Fig. 2.8a–c. Medial rotation splinting of left leg in the presence of joint laxity. **a** Left acetabulum more anteverted. **b** Left femur anteverted proximally. **c** X-ray confirms acetabular orientation. (Wilkinson 1963, with permission)

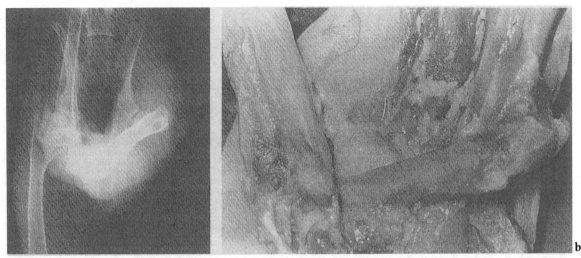

Fig. 2.10a,b. Hyperextension dislocation of the knee. The hip joint appears to be undisplaced radiologically. Note the medial rotation of the femoral shaft in the necropsy specimen. (Wilkinson 1963, with permission)

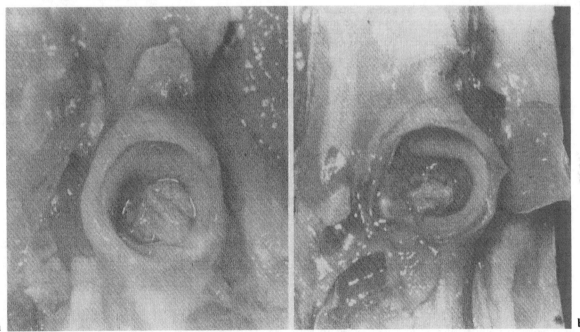

Fig. 2.11a,b. Intra-articular feature of anterior subluxation of left hip joint. Compare the normal appearance of the unsplinted right hip (a) and the medially splinted left hip (b). There is a loss of articular cartilage on the anterior third of the left acetabulum. (Wilkinson 1963, with permission)

of the hip joint. This was found to be infolded into the back of the joint and was revealed when the capsular ligament was opened anteriorly. The fold could be seen separating the femoral head from the posterior rim of the acetabulum. The ligamentum teres remained intact and had to be divided to reveal this feature of the posterior capsule. The posterior rim of the acetabulum also appeared to be worn away, suggesting that there had been some repeated posterior subluxation of the femoral head out of the acetabulum which had caused the stretching of the posterior capsule; in addition the lateral rotation of the hip had infolded the lax capsule into the joint to divide the cavity into a lateral compartment con-

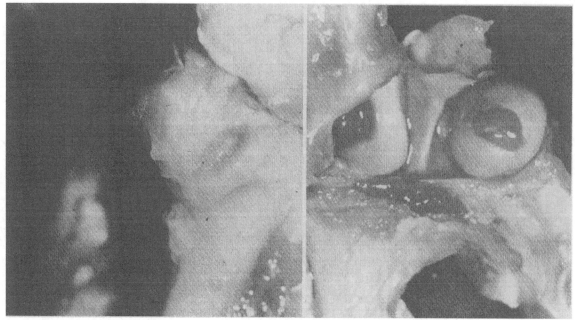

a   b

Fig. 2.12a,b. Posterior subluxation of male hip, resulting from a mild form of joint laxity and lateral rotation splinting. **a** Posterior aspect, revealing infolding of capsule. **b** Intra-articular appearance of posterior capsule, the femoral head being separated from the worn posterior rim by the infolded capsule.

taining the femoral head, and a separate medial retro-acetabular space, as seen in Fig. 2.12.

The conditioned *female* rabbits developed a more marked degree of generalised joint laxity which allowed the splints to be applied with minimal strain. Serial radiographs during the period of splinting showed the knees to flex, as the femurs rotated laterally. At necropsy a final X-ray revealed subluxation of the unsplinted hip joint because of the degree of capsular laxity; whereas on the splinted side, posterior dislocation of the hip had developed, associated with a shallowness of the acetabulum, due to a thickening of the bony floor, which appeared to extrude the femoral head and thus aggravated the displacement (Fig. 2.13).

Necropsy confirmed the posterior displacement of the femoral head with the lateral rotation of the femur, and incision of the anterior capsule revealed that the ligamentum teres was intact but elongated and thickened, allowing the femoral head to dislocate posteriorly, as shown in Fig. 2.14. When the ligamentum teres was divided, the posterior capsule again appeared to have an oblique white line dividing it into a lateral portion containing the femoral head and a medial retro-acetabular space. The posterior rim of the acetabulum was well worn by the repeated posterior displacements of the femoral head, shown in Fig. 2.15.

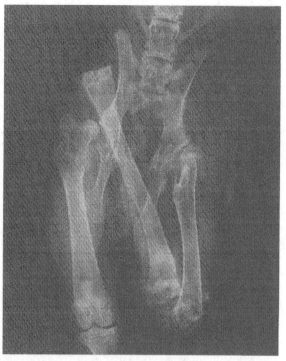

Fig. 2.13. Necropsy radiograph, female rabbit with hormonal laxity, subluxating right hip and dislocated left hip following lateral rotational splinting. Note the thickening of the floor of the left acetabulum, causing dysplasia and aggravating displacement. (Wilkinson 1963, with permission)

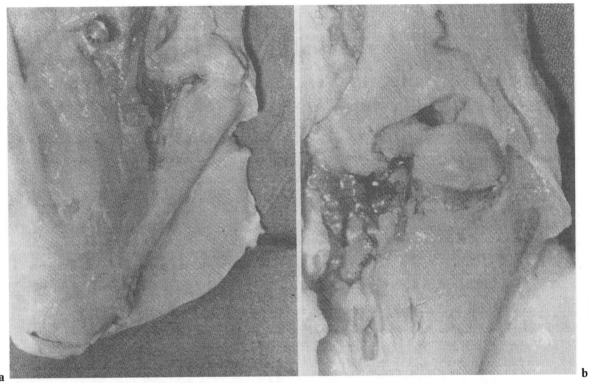

a   b

Fig. 2.14a,b. Experimental posterior dislocation, left hip. **a** Lateral rotation of flexed femur and flexed knee. **b** Thickened and elongated ligamentum teres. (Wilkinson 1963, with permission)

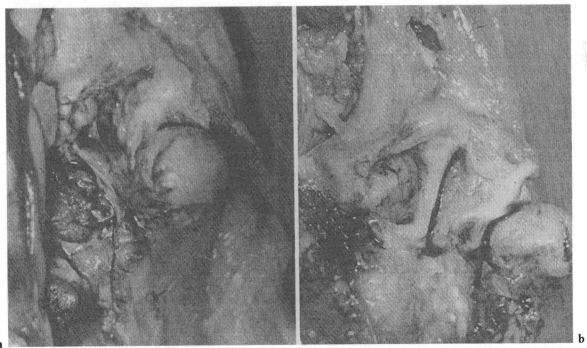

a   b

Fig. 2.15a,b. Experimental posterior dislocation left hip. **a** Ligamentum teres has been divided to reveal the main feature of the posterior capsule, an oblique white fold between the femoral head and acetabulum. **b** The white fold separates the lateral compartment containing the femoral head from the medial acetabular recess. (Wilkinson 1963, with permission)

In some specimens the anterior capsule had contracted and this appeared to prevent reduction of the femoral head into the acetabulum. The reduction was also impeded by the fold of posterior capsule lying between the femoral head and the posterior acetabular rim. Figure 2.16 is a diagrammatic summation of the soft tissue deformation with the hip flexed and looking down from above. The features include a contracture of the anterior capsule and a stretched and thickened ligamentum teres. The posterior capsule is stretched and infolded, dividing itself into a false lateral capsular acetabulum containing the femoral head and a medial retro-acetabular recess. The posterior labrum has been worn away. In none of these specimens was there any evidence of intra-articular haemorrhage or adhesion, as seen in the earlier experiments without hormonal injections. In the present series the intra-articular structures appear to be almost normal except for the described features. In all of these specimens, both male and female, the femurs were retroverted. Most of the deformity affected the proximal metaphysis. This was associated with retroversion of the acetabulum, as seen in Fig. 2.17.

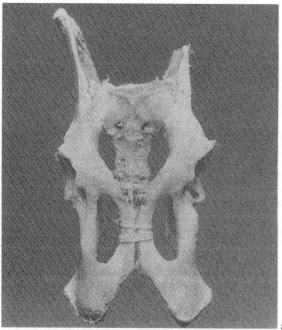

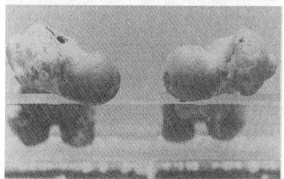

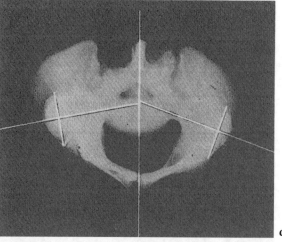

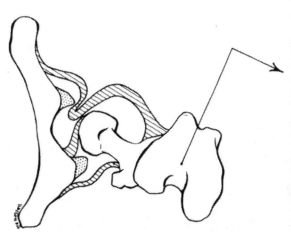

Fig. 2.16. Diagram of soft tissue deformation (see mirror image in Fig. 1.11), the lateral rotation of the flexed femur stretching the posterior capsule, and infolding it to form the limbus.

Fig. 2.17a–c. Lateral rotation splinting of left leg, in the presence of joint laxity. **a** Left acetabulum retroverted. **b** Left femur retroverted; note the femoral head is smaller, secondary to dislocation. **c** X-ray confirms acetabular orientation. (Wilkinson 1963, with permission)

Summary

Thus these experiments provided invaluable evidence to support the theory that environmental factors are responsible for posterior hip displacement, as they stress the combined effects of hormonal joint laxity and breech malposition in the pathogenesis of experimental atraumatic dislocation of the hip joint (Wilkinson 1963). They also provided the author with a complete understanding of similar anatomical features discovered later in the necropsy specimens of stillborn human foetuses, allowing him to comprehend their nature and the mechanism of their production.

References

Appleton AB (1934) Postural deformities and bone growth. Lancet 1:451

Arkin AM, Katz JF (1956) The effects of pressure on epiphyseal growth. J Bone Joint Surg 38A:1056

Dupuytren G (1847) Injuries and diseases of bones. Translated by F. Le Gros Clark for the Sydenham Society, London

Gill GG, Abbott LC (1942) Practical method of predicting the growth of the femur and tibia in the child. Arch Surg 17:380

Hall G (1981) Some observations of Perthes disease. J Bone Joint Surg 63B:631

Wilkinson JA (1962) Femoral anteversion in the rabbit. J Bone Joint Surg 44B:386

Wilkinson JA (1963) Prime factors in the etiology of congenital dislocation of the hip. J Bone Joint Surg 45B: 268

Wilkinson JA (1967) Experimental bone growth. J Bone Joint Surg 49B(3):583

3 Anatomy of Congenital Displacement of the Hip

Dissection of the stillborn foetus affords one insight into the early anatomical state.

J. Jackson Clarke (1910)

The only indisputable evidence concerning the effects of intra-uterine hormonal and mechanical factors on the pre-natal growth of the musculoskeletal system is seen in the variation of anatomical features found in the necropsy specimens of otherwise normal stillborn babies. Unfortunately our pathological museums do not provide many specimens for examination, so orthopaedic literature has few references and even those available fail to describe fully the soft tissue and bony components of the deformation.

Reference has already been made to the first description of congenital hip displacements in an 11-day-old boy made at necropsy by Paletta (1820; quoted by Trevor 1960), but details are not available in this case. Soon after Dupuytren (1847) described "original or congenital displacements of the heads of the thigh bones in patients reported to be quite healthy at birth". His evidence forced him to the conclusion that they were true congenital deformities and not the end result of foetal disease. He described 20 cases, but most were adults. Adolf Lorenz (1895) also contributed to the anatomical knowledge, but once again most of his observations were from surgery performed on older children.

Le Damany (1914) was probably the first to undertake extensive experimental and anatomical surveys. He dislocated the femoral heads of rabbit hip joints and compared the features of persistent dislocation to his detailed descriptions of soft tissue and bony features of the same deformity in human stillborns. Two main groups were recognised, including a rare teratological form of complete displacement and a commoner anthropologic deformation. He considered the latter to be uniquely human, believing it was caused by the longer thighs of the human foetus which needed excessive forms of folding in utero. He thought the long femurs produced torsional deformation of the hip joint resulting in acetabular changes and femoral anteversion during the last 3 months of pregnancy. These factors were responsible for anterior displacement of the hip joint when the hip extended. He described his own clinical test for hip instability (Dickson 1969) and found it to be commoner in girls.

In English literature, Jackson Clarke (1910) gave one of the earliest and most detailed monographs in which he described a specimen very accurately:

> The femoral head lay above but close to the acetabulum and the dislocation was easily reduced by inward rotation of the limb. The front part of the capsule was tense but the upper part became folded above the head and neck of the bone. The femoral head was flattened posteriorly and the ligamentum teres was elongated and flat. The cotyloid ligament was flattened against the upper part of the acetabulum.

There was "no serious degree of anteversion of the femoral neck" in any of his cases. Perhaps the greatest scientific contribution was made by Fairbank (1930) with a special reference to the anatomy at birth. His work and that of his colleague Ernest Hey Groves (1928) will be referred to later. Chandler (1929) also gave an accurate description of the intra-articular features found in the hips of an 11-day-old male infant who was born in the breech posture, with hyperextension dislocation of both knees and calcaneous moulding of both feet: "The thighs were laterally rotated. The hips were dislocated posteriorly and the femurs were retroverted."

Ortolani (1948) undertook extensive dissections upon stillborn foetal hips and made reference to Putti's original findings. He found modifications of the acetabular cavity evident in intra-uterine life, as seen in specimens from premature still births. They included a slight shallowing due to a "smoothing off" of the free border of the posterior portion of the fibrocartilaginous labrum. Changes in the angulation of the anatomical neck of the femur were not seen or were only minimal, leading him to believe that femoral anteversion represented a secondary modification. Ortolani believed that pre-natal deformation was minimal in the commoner form of "pre-luxation hip", when his snapping sign could be elicited. Later on, shortly after birth, the flattening of the labrum became accentuated and thickened and eventually acquired the characteristic shape of the external ear. He recognised a rarer form of pre-natal "luxation", which was confined to babies that had multiple malformations such as spina bifida and club feet. The femoral heads in all these hips were well-formed and were displaced into a wide secondary acetabulum, whereas the labrum was thickened and displaced downward, contributing to the reduction in size of the primary acetabulum, which was otherwise poorly developed. These he called "embryonary", pre-natal types of luxation and his snapping sign was rarely positive in such cases. The different conformation of these two groups was explained by the fact that "luxations", originating very early, were modified by the intra-uterine position of the foetus; but these features rarely developed in the later "pre-luxation" forms of displacement. Yet he found it impossible to make a clear distinction between the two forms of displacement.

A series of necropsy examinations were performed by the author on stillborn foetuses and on two babies who died cot-deaths within the first few weeks of life. Although the anatomical findings were described previously in 1962 (in his Robert Jones Essay, Hunterian Lecture and Thesis), the findings have not been published subsequently, because of the inclination of contemporary opinion to reject any theory of pre-natal deformation of the hip joint. The consensus of opinion has held that there is rarely any pre-natal deformity, and that the common form of congenital hip displacement consists of a simple laxity of the capsular ligaments at birth, so that this only leads to post-natal deformation in untreated cases. Four congenital subluxations and three congenital luxations have been discovered. The degrees of deformity affecting the soft tissues and bony components were related to the pregnancy history and birth postures in the majority of cases, and they have been compared with the anatomical features discovered in normal hip joints. With the information gained from experimental studies, described in Chap. 2, it has been possible to understand the nature of the deformity in most cases.

Normal Growth

If the hormonal and mechanical theories are to be confirmed, one should be able to identify the results of rotational strain placed on the flexed foetal hip and femur during functional development and growth, as seen in the three stages demonstrated in Fig. 3.1. Normally the foetus passes through the successive stages of intra-uterine posture to reach the final fully flexed posture before the 30th week. This means that the thighs then remain medially rotated, placing a similar rotational strain upon the femur and hip joint. In 10 full-term, stillborn babies delivered by cephalic presentation, necropsy revealed the common fully flexed cephalic posture. In every case the hips could be flexed, adducted and medially rotated without difficulty. The knees were also flexed and the feet moulded into valgus or varus position. All the femurs were found to be anteverted, the average measurement being 25°. The acetabula were also anteverted to the frontal position, their angles varying between 35° and 40° to the sagittal plane. The hip joints were stable and the intra-articular appearances were normal, with the surrounding labrum well-developed and clasping the femoral head, as shown in Fig. 3.2.

Abnormal Growth Due to Persistent Breech Malposition

There were nine stillborn breech births in the series, five being first-born females. These had normal hips and their femurs were anteverted. There were four male first-born breeches, whose legs were fully flexed at the hip joint and with semi-flexed knees that pointed laterally, as seen in Fig. 3.3. There was some restriction of medial rotation, but the hips

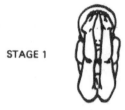

STAGE 1

BREECH POSTURE
12–26 weeks
UNIVERSAL PRIMARY POSTURE

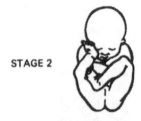

STAGE 2

FOLDING MECHANISM
26–32 weeks
PERSISTENCE OF THIS POSTURE PLACES
LATERAL TORSION ON THE FEMUR AND HIP
LEADING TO POSTERIOR DISLOCATION

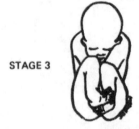

STAGE 3

VERTEX POSTURE
32–40 weeks
FINAL STABLE FULLY-FLEXED POSTURE

Fig. 3.1 The three stages of torsional malposition imposed on the foetal leg during normal development. Stage 1: medial rotation. Stage 2: lateral rotation. Stage 3: medial rotation, on the flexed hip. The period of time in each stage is maximal. (Wilkinson 1966, with permission)

were undisplaced. The intra-articular architecture appeared to be normal and the labrum was well-developed, surrounding the femoral head in each hip joint. The acetabula were more laterally placed, and the angle from the sagittal line averaged approximately 50°. The femurs were also retroverted.

All the anatomical features described above were considered to be within the limits of normal development, with normal intra-articular architecture of the hip joints; the bony components ranged from anteverted femurs and acetabula associated with the cephalic posture, to the more retroverted femurs and laterally placed acetabula associated with the lateral rotation breech posture. It was interesting to note that there was less bony deformation associated with the more lax female joints, as compared to the males.

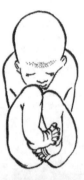

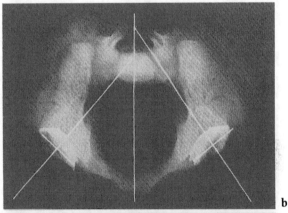

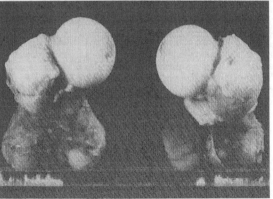

Fig. 3.2a–c. Final, fully-flexed foetal posture. **a** Preceding cephalic version. Hips flexed, adducted and medially rotated (Wilkinson 1966, with permission). **b** Acetabular anteversion: 35°–40° to sagittal plane. **c** Femurs anteverted 25°, enabling the new-born to extend and medially rotate the thighs without subluxating the hip joints.

28

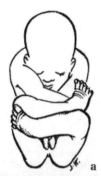

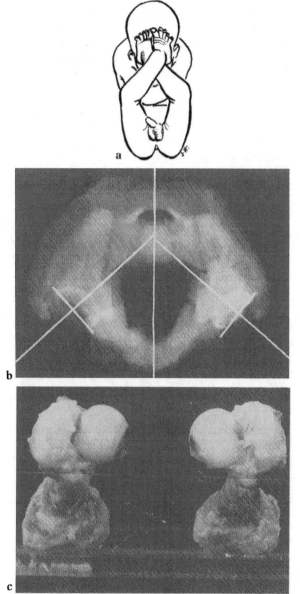

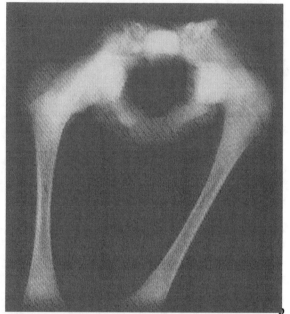

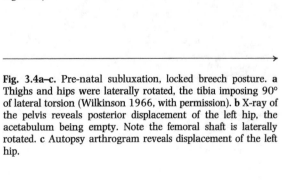

Fig. 3.3a–c. Lateral rotation breech posture. **a** Semi-flexed knees and thighs laterally rotated (Wilkinson 1966, with permission). **b** Acetabula laterally rotated 50° from sagittal line. **c** Femurs are retroverted. Postural extension and medial rotation of the thighs would tend to displace the femoral heads posteriorly (see Fig. 3.20).

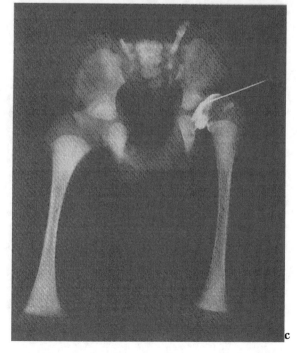

Fig. 3.4a–c. Pre-natal subluxation, locked breech posture. **a** Thighs and hips were laterally rotated, the tibia imposing 90° of lateral torsion (Wilkinson 1966, with permission). **b** X-ray of the pelvis reveals posterior displacement of the left hip, the acetabulum being empty. Note the femoral shaft is laterally rotated. **c** Autopsy arthrogram reveals displacement of the left hip.

Pre-natal Subluxations

In some of the female stillborns wrapped in the lateral rotation breech posture, abnormal intra-articular features were found in varying degrees. Their legs could be easily placed in the locked breech posture with 90° of lateral rotation and there was usually an associated valgus moulding of both feet, the posture being demonstrated in Fig. 3.4.

Some of the hip joints were unstable and posterior displacement was demonstrated by autopsy arthrograms. The intra-articular structure appeared to be normal at first, as the ligamentum teres was always intact, but elongated to a sufficient length to allow posterior displacement. When divided, the posterior capsule was found to be thickened, stretched, and inverted. The posterior labrum was worn away, from the repeated posterior displacements, as seen in Fig. 3.5.

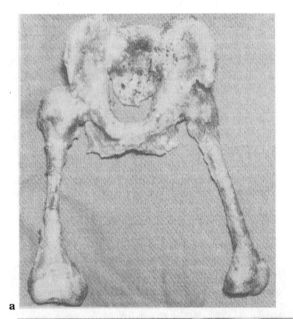
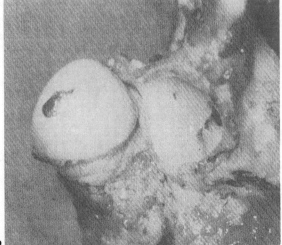
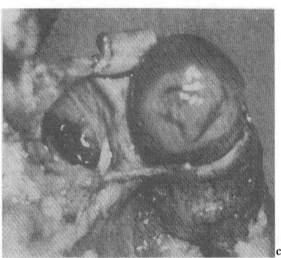

Fig. 3.5a–c. Pre-natal subluxation, soft tissue features. **a** Left hip displacement: note lateral rotation of femur (Wilkinson 1966, with permission). **b** Normal intra-articular structure of right hip. **c** Left subluxation. Ligamentum teres has been divided to reveal posterior capsule, thickened, stretched and inverted. Note that the labrum has been worn away by recurrent posterior displacement (see Fig. 2.12).

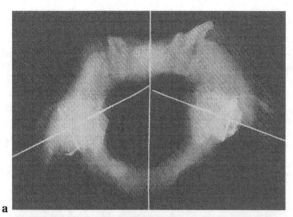

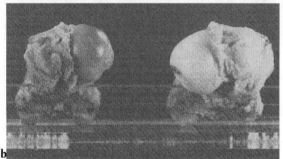

Fig. 3.6a,b. Deformation of bony components in pre-natal subluxation. **a** The pelvis with a more laterally rotated shallow acetabulum, due to the thickening of the bony floor. **b** Femoral retroversion; note the left femoral head is smaller secondary to displacement, but less retroverted than the non-displaced side (see Fig. 2.17).

The femurs were always retroverted, especially on the non-dislocated side, and the displaced femoral head usually appeared smaller than the normal. The acetabulum was more retroverted than on the non-dislocated side, and the floor of the acetabulum appeared thicker than the normal. This made the acetabular cavity appear shallow, as seen in Fig. 3.6.

Pre-natal Luxations

There was a specimen from a stillborn male, the result of a 30-week pregnancy, terminating in a frank breech left footling presentation. The stillborn appeared normal from external examination and the birth death was due to cerebral trauma. The legs were very lax and could be placed easily in the locked breech posture. The left foot was oedematous and blue due to its previous presentation. There did not appear to be any leg-shortening and both hips abducted fully. Dissection however revealed a complete congenital displacement on the right side. The

femoral head was contained in a false acetabulum consisting of a thickened capsule and was separated from the original acetabulum by a crescentic limbus extending over the superior, posterior, and inferior aspects of the acetabular rim, seen in Fig. 3.7. The ligamentum teres was intact and could be traced from the femoral head to the site of the true bony acetabulum. The infolding of the posterior capsule formed an oblique obstruction lying between the false capsule containing the femoral head and the retro-acetabular recess. The appearance was originally described by Sir Thomas Fairbank (1930) in his monumental contribution to the understanding of the anatomy of congenital dislocation of the hip, in which he stated,

... there is a fold which lies more or less horizontally, but is inclined downwards. It is soft and not cartilaginous and is in fact a fold of synovial membrane and posterior capsule. It helps to divide the cavity of the joint into three portions, the old acetabulum, the retroacetabular space and the false acetabulum. During manipulative reduction the fold is piled up onto the acetabular margin and increases the difficulty in forcing the femoral head to traverse the second compartment on its way from the third to the first. As the head migrates

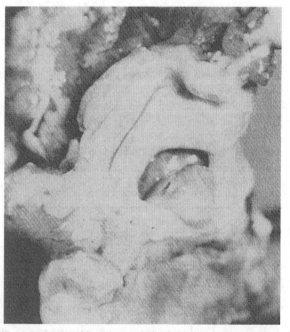

Fig. 3.7. Pre-natal luxation, right hip. There is a crescentic limbus extending along the superior, posterior, and inferior segments. The divided ligamentum teres can be seen to emerge from the bony acetabulum, through the hiatus bounded by the limbus.

it carries in front of it a dome of the capsule which blends with the periosteum above and behind the acetabulum.

Thus, in this specimen the retro-acetabular recess had disappeared and the fold of the posterior capsule had become adherent to the posterior rim of the acetabulum. In this hip joint the anterior capsule had contracted, and this also prevented a reduction of the femoral head by restricting the degree of abduction, thus stabilising the permanent displacement of the femoral head. When the anterior capsule and ligamentum teres were divided the limbus could be seen surrounding the superior, posterior, and inferior aspects of the acetabulum and encroaching upon its access. Cross-sections of such specimens, stained to highlight the collagenous fibres, revealed the thickened posterior capsule infolded and adherent to the back of the cartilaginous acetabulum, obliterating the retro-

acetabular recess (which is clearly defined at birth in the normal hip joint), as seen in Fig. 3.8.

Pathological Luxations

A specimen of bilateral hip displacement was obtained from a stillborn with a severe degree of arthrogryphosis affecting both upper and lower limbs. It was a full-term male child, breech born, but died within $7\frac{1}{2}$ h of birth. The locked breech posture had been imposed upon the legs, which were held rigidly with both hips and knees flexed, though the thighs were laterally rotated 90°. It was not possible to correct, passively, the fixed deformities of the hips and knees. Both feet were clubbed and all the affected joints were quite stiff.

The pelvis and hips were removed and X-rayed; the films confirmed a bilateral posterior displacement of the femoral heads with a severe degree of

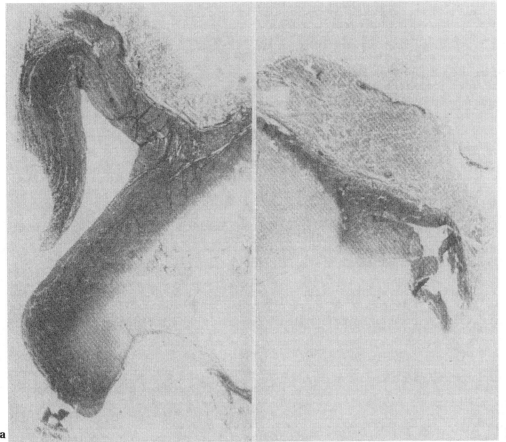

a   b

Fig. 3.8a,b. Pre-natal luxation, right hip. **a** The thickened posterior capsule is infolded, and the fold is adherent to the posterior aspect of the cartilaginous acetabulum obliterating the retro-acetabular recess. **b** The left hip is normal. Note the labrum is separated from the capsule by the retro-acetabular recess.

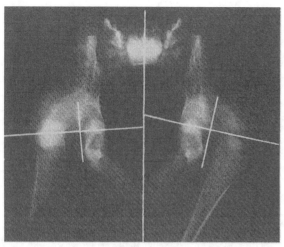

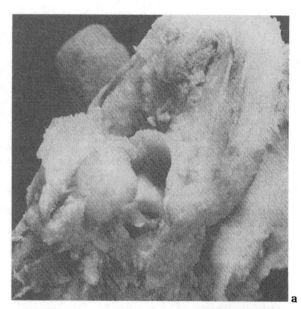

Fig. 3.9. Arthrogryphosis with bilateral pre-natal luxations. The femoral heads are displaced posteriorly and the acetabula are faced laterally.

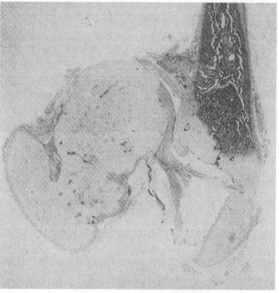

retroversion of both acetabula (Fig. 3.9). Dissection of the hips revealed complete posterior displacement of both femoral heads, each of which was contained in a false acetabulum consisting of a thickened posterior capsule, but separated from the true bony acetabulum by an intervening limbus. The latter formed a complete obstruction to the reduction of the femoral head, leaving only a small hiatus for the intact ligamentum teres to penetrate and extend to the base of the acetabular floor, as shown in Fig. 3.10.

Cross-sections of the left hip revealed the limbus to be a fold of posterior capsule adhering to the posterior rim of the acetabulum. The retro-acetabular recess had been obliterated and the femoral head was contained in the false capsular acetabulum. The femoral head itself was cartilaginous, but contained vascular sinusoids.

These congenital hip displacements were secondary to the pathological muscle imbalance of the generalised arthrogryphosis. This had interfered with the folding mechanism of the legs in early foetal development, resulting in the same intra-articular features as seen in those pre-natal luxations found in otherwise normal stillborns.

Fig. 3.10a,b. Arthrogryphosis, pre-natal luxation. **a** Femoral head contained in false acetabulum, the ligamentum teres stretching to the true bony acetabulum. Note the extent of the limbus. **b** Cross-section of the luxation, the femoral head being contained in the false capsular acetabulum and separated by the infolded capsule from the true acetabulum. Note the ligamentum teres.

Congenital Displacement of the Knee and Hip Joint

Although the usual mechanism of intra-uterine hip displacement is as previously described, there is another mechanism which is rare. It involves medial rotation of the hips with hyperextension of the knee joints. This mechanism is more prone to produce pre-natal hyperextension dislocation of the knee joint; the hip usually remains stable, as was discovered in the animal experiments described in Chap. 2 (see Fig. 2.10).

According to Tubby (1912) a review of 121 cases of congenital dislocation of the knee (CDK) was previously performed by Tridon (1905), and he discovered that only 20 of these patients had an associated CDH. The author came to the conclusion that the bulk of cases of CDK were due to intra-uterine mechanical causes. Thus it appears that the medial rotation breech posture is more likely to produce hyperextension CDK than CDH, but the latter does occur.

In my long series over the past 25 years, there have been three patients with the combined congenital dislocation of the knee and hip joints. In each case the knees responded to simple flexion splinting at birth. In one the hips stabilised spontaneously but in the other two patients the hips were reduced by delayed open surgery with good results (Fig. 3.11).

The Development of CDH

The mechanism of posterior displacement of the femoral head over the posterior rim of the acetabulum in the flexed hip posture was described in Chap. 1. Such a displacement can only occur when there is a laxity of the capsular ligament, the product of mechanical stretching and a hormonal influence or genetic factors. Such a mechanism produces retroversion of the femur and acetabulum. These bony features allow the flexed hip to assume the position of lateral rotation, when there is not enough laxity of the capsular ligament to facilitate displacement.

Soft Tissue Deformation

The first stage of displacement involves the stretching of the capsule and ligamentum teres by the recurrent rotational displacement of the femoral head over the rim of the acetabulum. This mechanism also wears away the posterior labrum. Such a degree of deformation is called a "pre-natal subluxation", as there is no impediment to spontaneous concentric reduction of the femoral head when the leg is either abducted in neutral rotation or extended and laterally rotated. Thus the majority of these unstable hips undergo spontaneous and complete recovery. Figure 3.12 represents the degree of displacement and illustrates its concentric reduction.

There is a second stage of displacement and soft tissue deformation produced by the same mechanism. Recurrent rotational displacement of the femoral head initially stretches the posterior capsule and later infolds it into the joint. This fold divides the posterior capsule into a larger lateral portion containing the femoral head and a smaller medial

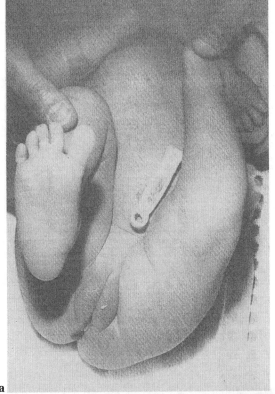

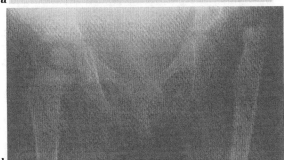

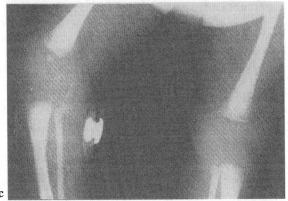

Fig. 3.11a–c. Congenital displacement of knees and hips. **a** Newborn with hyperextension dislocation of left knee. **b** Left hip is displaced. **c** Left knee—hyperextension dislocation. Absent distal femoral epiphysis.

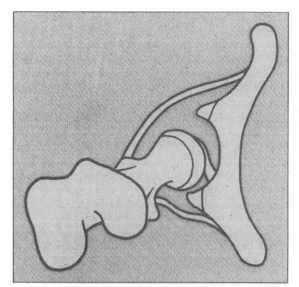

Fig. 3.12. Pre-natal subluxation. The stretched posterior capsule and ligamentum teres allow recurrent posterior displacement of the femoral head, causing the wearing away of the posterior labrum.

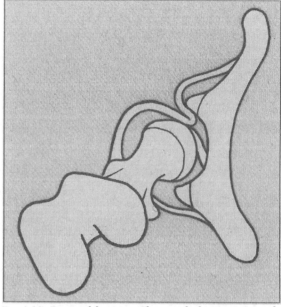

Fig. 3.13. Pre-natal luxation. The stretched posterior capsule has infolded to divide itself into a lateral compartment containing the femoral head and a retro-acetabular recess.

retro-acetabular recess. Eventually the fold becomes adherent to the worn posterior rim of the acetabulum, thus obliterating the retro-acetabular recess. In this way it comes to form an obstruction lying between the femoral head and the acetabulum. This prevents spontaneous reduction of the displacement. Later the anterior capsule contracts and this finally stabilises the complete displacement of the femoral head. This degree of displacement is called a "pre-natal luxation" and it is illustrated in Fig. 3.13.

Thus there are two degrees of CDH at birth. The commoner form is that in which there is a combination of capsular laxity with increased retroversion of the two bony components. The laxity allows the femoral head to slip in and out of the acetabulum providing a clear "clunk" on reduction, which is the basis of the positive Ortolani sign. Concentric reduction can occur and the disappearance of hormonal laxity usually stabilises the joint. Thus spontaneous recovery is high and many such hips escape diagnosis.

The rarer form of CDH at birth has a second stage of deformation with an infolded posterior capsule, which might well become incarcerated into the acetabulum. This prevents concentric reduction, causing a negative Ortolani sign, or a "muffled" clunk which might be missed on clinical examination, except by the most vigilant observers. Spontaneous reduction in these cases is unlikely to occur, and that means that the displacement might well

persist into infant life to be diagnosed when the child begins to walk.

These two degrees of CDH at birth are illustrated in Fig. 3.14.

This is where orthopaedic opinion still remains divided, because there are those who believe that all cases of CDH have no soft tissue deformation at birth other than capsular laxity. Thus these authorities uphold that there can be no impediment to reduction and diagnosis is evident in most cases at birth. As they accept that all CDH can be reduced concentrically, simple splinting at birth must cure most patients!

However, it is becoming increasingly recognised that the second stage of deformity may well be present at birth. In these patients enforced abduction splinting might cause pressure necrosis of the bony components due to eccentric reduction of the hip. In these cases diagnosis can be very difficult and spontaneous recovery is unlikely to take place, because of the incarceration of the infolded posterior capsule, or limbus.

Peter Dunn (1976) in a large series of perinatal autopsies collected 47 congenitally displaced hip joints in 31 babies, of which 50% were breech born, the gestation ages ranging from 27 to 44 weeks. He divided his specimens of dislocatable hips into three grades, ranging from the mildest form of soft tissue deformation in Grade 1, to a complete dislocation

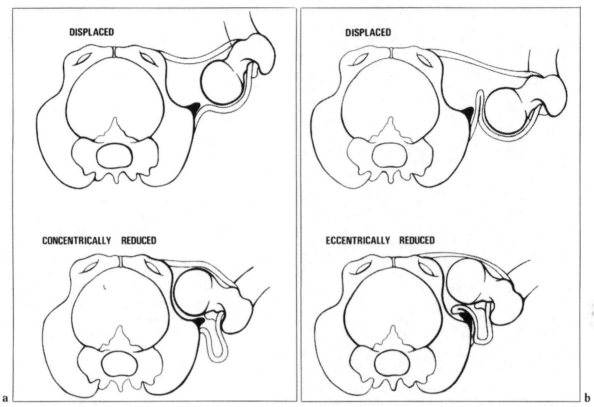

Fig. 3.14a,b. Unstable new-born hip, without and with a limbus. **a** Simple laxity of capsule and ligamentum teres, allowing posterior displacement and concentric reduction. **b** Posterior capsule infolded to form a limbus, preventing concentric reduction. (Wilkinson 1972, with permission)

in Grade 3. There appeared to be "a spectrum of severity in a single pathological process" and he defined CDH as "an anomaly of the hip joint present at birth in which the head of the femur is, as may be, partially or completely dislocated from the acetabulum". Dunn estimated that 1% of all new-borns in the United Kingdom have CDH, and of these, 85% are otherwise normally formed; among the latter, 90% are Grade 1 (pre-natal subluxation) and 10% are Grade 2 or 3 (complete displacements), being the near equivalent of one in a thousand normal live births.

Thus, although many authorities would have us believe that pre-natal congenital luxation is a rare deformity and frequently associated with multiple deformities, there is overwhelming evidence to show that the deformation is not uncommon in otherwise normally developed new-borns. Increasing degrees of soft tissue deformation evolve pre-natally, and even Ortolani himself had difficulty in making a clear distinction between the two forms of displacement.

Bone Deformation

In all these specimens of lateral rotation breech posture with hip displacement, the femoral head on the affected side was smaller than the normal and in addition the femoral neck was more retroverted than normal; the acetabulum was also more retroverted in relation to the sagittal plane and the socket appeared shallow owing to a thickening of the bony floor. In other words, the depth of the acetabulum was inadequate and there was, as Henry Jacob Biglow of Harvard described in 1844, "a rising up of the bottom of the socket, which seems to result from the absence of pressure" (Hart 1948; see Fig. 3.15).

Ernest Hey Groves (1928) in his classic contribution to the Robert Jones Birthday Volume, based his surgical management of congenital dislocation of the hip on the firm foundation of his understanding of normal and pathological anatomy. He had no difficulty in collecting adult specimens, but could find

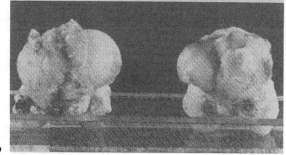

a

b

Fig. 3.15a,b. Bony components of pre-natal luxation, right hip.
a X-ray of acetabula revealing soft tissue features and thickened
bony floor of right acetabulum. **b** Femurs: the right femoral head
is smaller, conical in shape and retroverted.

only one specimen from a full-term, male, stillborn which was kept in the Hunterian Museum of the Royal College of Surgeons, England, illustrated in Fig. 3.16.

His drawings revealed a pre-natal luxation with the femoral head contained in a false capsular acetabulum, being separated from the original acetabulum by a circumferential limbus only penetrated by an intact ligamentum teres. The obstruction was called a "cotyloid ligament". The acetabulum was described as shallow, whereas the head and the greater trochanter of the dislocated femur appeared smaller than normal and the head was of conical form. Fortunately, the specimen survived the wartime blitz of the Royal College, and in recognition of its identification, the author was allowed to dismount and photograph the pelvis and femur (Fig. 3.17). It can be seen that the femoral head is retroverted, the bony deformation being a record of the previously existing breech malposition that had imposed a lateral rotational strain upon the foetal hip joint resulting in its posterior displacement, as well as the soft tissue deformation and the retroversion of the bony acetabulum. Little did the Master realise that the very key to its "mysterious origin" lay in his hands.

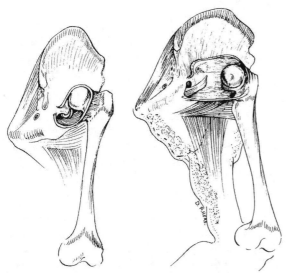

Fig. 3.16. Illustration of CDH in stillborn. (Hey Groves 1928, with permission)

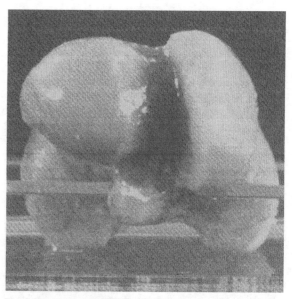

Fig. 3.17. Femur of CDH in stillborn. Note that it is retroverted. (Hey Groves' specimen, RCS)

Post-natal Development

When new-borns survive the challenge of birth, very few succumb to disease and therefore the numbers of post-natal specimens of congenital hip displacement remain scarce. Thus the understanding of the biomechanical changes that take place in early neonatal and later infantile life must be based largely on conjecture, backed up by clinical and surgical findings. The latter however have proved to be misleading in the past, because of the limited surgical approach to such a complex biomechanical problem.

It must be remembered that the hip joint never extends in utero, but is kept in a fully flexed posture. Weinberg and Pogrund (1980) have recently pointed out that in order to attain this intra-uterine posture, the pelvis must be rotated in an anticlockwise direction in the sagittal plane until the iliac crests point posteriorly, thus making the iliac portion of the acetabulum its posterior rim. Soon after birth extension of the spine, pelvis and hip joints produces a derotation of the acetabulum through 90° in a

clockwise direction, bringing the iliac portion of the acetabular rim into the superior area of the socket. Thus the intra-uterine mechanism of posterior hip displacement involves the repetitive sliding of the femoral head over the iliac portion of the acetabular rim. Later the structural changes observed in the stillborn specimens, affecting the posterior rim of the acetabulum, are rotated superiorly to the future weight-bearing area, as demonstrated in Fig. 3.18.

This torsional effect upon the hip joint is reflected in the structure of the capsular ligaments, the fibres of which run in a clockwise direction. In utero, the capsular fibres stretch between the posterior aspect of the acetabulum to the anterior aspect of the femoral neck. Post-natally, when the hip joint has rotated through a 90° arc in a clockwise direction, the same fibres run from the posterior aspect of the acetabulum over the summit of the femoral head to the anterior aspect of the femoral neck; whereas the fibres arising from the anterior part of the acetabulum are inserted posteriorly into the intertrochanteric crest, as seen in Fig. 3.19.

The unfolding of the pelvis in a clockwise direction also affects the rotational stability of the hip joint. It has been seen in the normal hips of full-term,

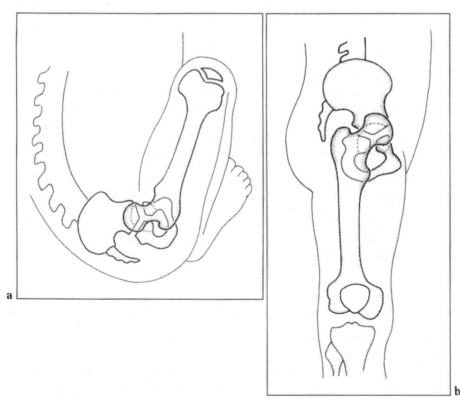

Fig. 3.18a,b. Pre-natal anticlockwise and post-natal clockwise rotation of the pelvis. **a** Pre-natally the ilium lies horizontally and the femoral head displaces over this part of the acetabular rim. **b** Post-natally the ilium rotates 90° to a vertical position and the instability is aggravated by the extension and lateral rotation of the femur.

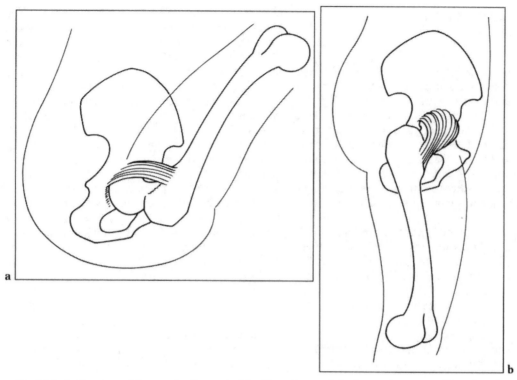

Fig. 3.19a,b. Structure of the capsular ligament of the hip. **a** Pre-natal development—posterior fibres span from the back of the acetabulum to the front of the femur. **b** Post-natal extension stretches these fibres over the summit of the hip joint, in a clockwise direction.

cephalic-delivered stillborns that the acetabula and femurs are anteverted. This allows the new-born freedom to extend and medially rotate the legs without placing any strain on the hips. In the breech-born babies with more retroverted acetabula and femurs, the bony components of the hip are congruous in the flexed and abducted posture; but when the legs are extended and medially rotated, the retroverted femoral head tends to displace posteriorly, aggravating any instability of the joint due to laxity of the capsule. This is the basis of Andren's radiological test (1961), in which hip instability is revealed by extending, abducting, and medially rotating the infant's legs. This manoeuvre tends to displace the femoral head, according to the degree of femoral retroversion and joint laxity. Thus in breech births, it is dangerous to force the new-born baby's legs into extension and medial rotation, and one has to wait for the gradual development of acetabular and femoral anteversion brought about by the gradual medial rotation and extension of the thighs, as demonstrated in Fig. 3.20.

On three occasions, cot-deaths have provided specimens of congenital hip displacement that were detected after birth, the diagnosis being made by the presence of positive Ortolani tests. It was not surprising to find in the specimens that the intra-articular appearances were quite normal, as these were cases of pre-natal subluxation. After the division of the intact ligamentum teres, the posterior labrum was usually found to be worn away and this was associated with a slight infolding of the lax posterior capsule; the femurs and acetabula were retroverted more than the normal, as shown in Fig. 3.21.

Neonatal Congenital Displacement

When the congenital displacement is complete and the femoral head is prevented from entering the bony acetabulum because of the presence of the limbus, standing and walking will cause the thigh to rotate medially and the femur becomes anteverted owing to the medial rotational torsion placed upon it. This force is not transmitted to the acetabulum, because of the persistent displacement and the laxity of the capsule, and so it remains retroverted. Such a combination of femoral anteversion and acetabular retroversion led to the misunderstanding that the primary displacement was anterior.

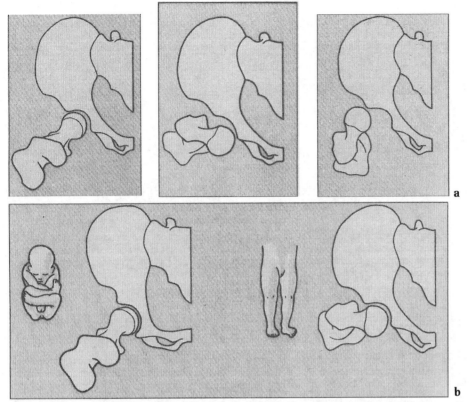

Fig. 3.20a,b. Post-natal hip instability and stability. **a** In hip displacement, retroversion of the femur and acetabulum are congruous in flexion and lateral rotation, and in extension and lateral rotation. Hip extension and medial rotation (Andren's test) produces posterior displacement, when capsular laxity is present. **b** In the absence of capsular laxity, the locked breech posture can only be assumed when both bony components are retroverted. Similarly, postural extension and medial rotation of the hips can only be assumed when anteversion develops in the two bony components.

Only one specimen has been collected in this series, as such acquisition is dependent upon a concomitant fatal disease in infancy. A girl child with generalised joint laxity was known to have been born with instability of her left hip, there being a positive Ortolani sign at birth. She suffered from Von Gierke's disease and died at the age of 7 months. Because of her weak condition her CDH was never splinted, but she was encouraged to sit up with her legs extended and medially rotated. An X-ray taken just before death revealed persistent dysplasia of the left hip with some degree of subluxation. A necropsy arthrogram with both femurs flexed and abducted revealed a contracture of the anterior capsule limiting abduction on the left side. It could also be seen that the left acetabulum was more sagittally placed than the right and the bony floor was thicker on the left than the right side (Ralis and McKibbin 1973), as seen in Fig. 3.22.

The intra-articular structures first appeared normal, but when the ligamentum teres was divided, the posterior capsule of the left hip was thickened and infolded. Examination of the bony components revealed that the left acetabulum was shallower; this was partly due to the thickened bony floor, but also it was more sagittal than the right, the angle to the sagittal plane being nearly 10° greater. Both femurs were anteverted, but the torsion appeared to affect the distal third of the femoral shafts and not the proximal metaphysis, suggesting that it might well have occurred post-natally due to the posture of the lower limbs during the 7 months of life.

Structure and Blood Supply to the Femoral Head

At birth the femoral head consists of pre-osseous cartilage and has been described to be rather like india rubber, being resilient but compressible (Salter et al. 1969). Its precarious blood supply has been

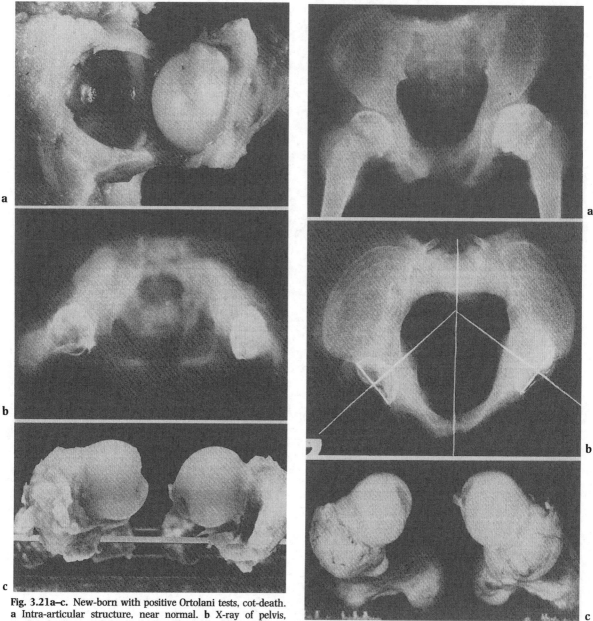

Fig. 3.21a–c. New-born with positive Ortolani tests, cot-death. a Intra-articular structure, near normal. b X-ray of pelvis, necropsy arthrogram, retroversion of both acetabula. c Both femurs were retroverted.

Fig. 3.22a–c. Neonatal congenital dislocation (left). a Necropsy arthrograms in forced flexion and abduction. Note the contracture of anterior capsule left hip and central pooling of dye. b X-ray of pelvis—left acetabulum shallow partly due to thickened bony floor, and more retroverted than right. c Femurs. Left head smaller due to displacement, femoral heads retroverted, but shafts are anteverted distally (post-natal).

recorded in intimate detail by many authorities. One of the earliest contributions was made by Astley Cooper (1822), but our present day concept is based on the work of Tucker (1949) and Trueta (1957), whose theories have not been challenged.

The capital blood supply, at birth, is mainly dependent upon the metaphyseal branches of the nutrient artery and they run upward from the ossifying border of the diaphysis through the cartila-

ginous head. They form sinusoids in the cartilage and there is very little anastomosis. Even the slightest pressure can obliterate them. A second supply is provided by the lateral epiphyseal vessels which run at right angles to these metaphyseal branches and the former are responsible for the eventual ossification of the femoral head. The vessels in the ligamentum teres are least important, although they do penetrate the femoral head. There is no anastomosis between the three systems and all are exposed to any pressure placed upon the femoral head. Perhaps the metaphyseal vessels are at greatest risk, as they can be compressed up against the ossified diaphysis. The arrangement persists up to the fourth month, and during this initial period the proximal femoral growth is at greatest risk. Even the slightest compression can produce infarction, which is more likely to affect the cartilaginous precursor of the epiphyseal growth plate before the pre-osseous cartilage of the epiphysis due to its juxtadiaphyseal position.

At 4 months the penetrating vessels from the ligamentum teres disappear and this coincides with the appearance of the secondary ossific centre in the femoral head, and the constitution of the epiphyseal plate. The metaphyseal vessels become cut off by the development of the physis, making the lateral epiphyseal vessels totally responsible for its supply and also that to the epiphyseal nucleus. As the epiphysis develops between the fourth and the eighteenth months its osseous structure hardens and protects the epiphyseal blood supply from any pressure.

In a personal communication (1980), Graham Hall conveyed the results of his load-bearing experiments on immature pigs' hips. He removed the

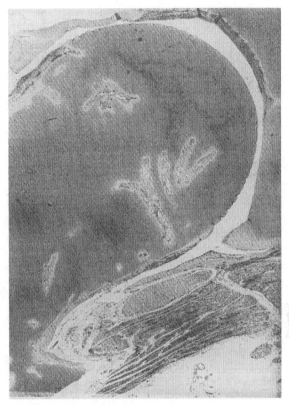

Fig. 3.23. Femoral head at birth, consisting of hyaline cartilage "rather like india-rubber, being resilient, but compressible". Note the sinusoids, few and isolated.

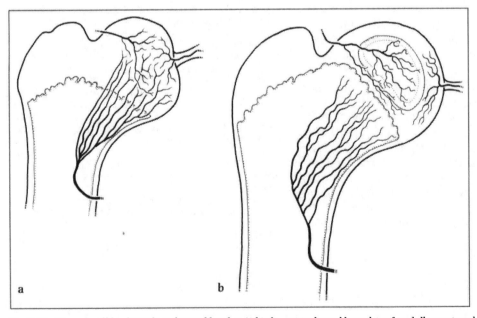

Fig. 3.24. Diagram of blood supply to femoral head. **a** At birth—metaphyseal branches of medullary artery, lateral epiphyseal vessels and arterioles in ligamentum teres. **b** At 10 months, the appearance of the epiphysis and physis cut off the metaphyseal branch. The lateral and, to a lesser extent, the medial epiphyseal vessels become totally responsible for the blood supply.

femoral heads of immature pigs within 24 h of death, from two groups. The first group were still-born piglets where the ossific nucleus had not developed, and the second group were 6-month-old pigs, where the ossific nucleus occupied 60% of the volume of the cartilaginous femoral head. Increasing loads were applied to each hip until mechanical failure occurred. For a given load the hip of the still-born piglet, which is totally cartilaginous, deforms by a relatively greater amount than that of a hip in which there is an ossific nucleus. Hall came to the conclusion that a totally cartilaginous hip deforms under load by approximately twice the amount of one with an ossific nucleus occupying 60% of the hip's volume. The presence of an ossific nucleus greatly increased the mechanical strength of the hip.

Summary

Thus the indisputable evidence concerning the effects of intra-uterine hormonal and mechanical factors on the pre-natal growth of the musculo-skeletal system indicates:

1) That normal foetal growth is dependent upon intrinsic embryological, genetic, and hormonal factors, but is also influenced by extrinsic maternal hormones and intra-uterine mechanical factors.

2) Abnormal foetal growth is usually due to an exaggerated influence of these extrinsic factors causing a delay in normal functional development.

3) Persistent lateral rotation breech malposition clearly influences the flexed foetal hip, producing soft tissue and bony deformation in varying degrees.

4) Two stages of posterior hip displacement have been identified at birth. A spectrum of changes separate the two extremes from a simple laxity of the capsular ligaments, to a complete inversion of the stretched posterior capsule causing a total impediment to the spontaneous replacement of the femoral head.

5) Post-natal growth is influenced by extension of the hip joint for the first time; this distorts the soft tissues and also produces torsional changes in the bony components. At the same time there are changes in the consistency and viability of the femoral head, brought about by the development of the proximal femoral epiphysis.

References

Andren L (1961) Aetiology and diagnosis of congenital dislocation of the hip in newborns. Radiologe 1:89–94

Chandler FA (1929) Congenital dislocation of the hip. An anatomical study of a case of bilateral C.D.H. and other associated deformities. J Bone Joint Surg 11:546–556

Clarke, JJ (1910) Congenital dislocation of the hip. Ballière, Tindall & Cox, London

Cooper A (1822) A treatise on dislocation and fractures of the joints. Longman, London

Dickson J (1969) Pierre Le Damany on congenital dysplasia of the hip. Proc R Soc Med 62:575

Dunn P (1976) Perinatal observations on the aetiology of congenital dislocation of the hip. Clin Orthop 119:11

Dupuytren G (1847) Injuries and diseases of bones. Translated by F. Le Gros Clark for the Sydenham Society, London

Fairbank T (1930) Congenital dislocation of the hip with special reference to anatomy. Br J Surg 17:380

Hart VL (1948) Congenital dysplasia of the hip joint and sequelae. Charles E. Thomas, Illinois

Hey Groves E (1928) The treatment of congenital dislocation of the hip. Robert Jones Birthday Volume, Oxford University Press, Oxford

Le Damany P (1914) Congenital luxation of the hip. Am J Orthop Surg 11(4):541

Lorenz A (1896) Care of congenital luxation of the hip by bloodless reduction and weighting. Trans Am Orthop Assoc 9:254

Ortolani M (1948) La lussazione congenita dell'anca—Nuovi criteri diagnostici e profilattico-correttivi. Cappelli, Bologna

Ralis ZA, McKibbin B (1973) Changes in shape of the human hip joint during its development and their relation to its stability. J Bone Joint Surg 55B(4):780–785

Salter RB, Kostuick J, Dallas S (1969) Avascular necrosis of the femoral head as a complication of treatment of C.D.H. in young children. Can J Surg 12:44

Trevor D (1960) Treatment of congenital hip dysplasia in older children. Proc R Soc Med 53:481

Trueta J (1957) The normal vascularity of the human femoral head during growth. J Bone Joint Surg 39B:358

Tucker F (1949) Arterial supply to the femoral head and its clinical importance. J Bone Joint Surg 31B:82

Weinberg H, Pogrund H (1980) Effect of pelvic inclination on the pathogenesis of congenital hip dislocation. Isr J Med Sci 16(4):229–233

Wilkinson JA (1972) A post-natal survey for congenital dislocation of the hip. J Bone Joint Surg 54B:40

4 Genetic and Environmental Aetiological Factors and Family Studies in the Prevalence of CDH

One can classify normal human variations into that which is mostly due to genetic difference, that which is mostly due to differing environmental experience, and that which is a combination of both genetic and environmental difference.

C. O. Carter (1962)

Usually CDH affects normal children and like most instances of common congenital deformation it has a mixed developmental and environmental aetiology. Although the details of neither group are fully established, twin studies demonstrate the importance of these factors.

Idelberger in 1951 in his large survey of twins from southern Germany found that when one twin had a congenital displacement, 34% of monozygotic or identical co-twins were similarly affected, as compared with only 3% of dizygotic or non-identical co-twins. This last figure is no greater than the incidence among sisters and brothers of patients with CDH, indicating that the twin pregnancy itself does not provide a mechanical factor. It is also confirmed by the fact that there was no increase in the prevalence of the condition among twin births in the population.

The finding that identical uni-ovular twins are significantly affected, as compared with non-identical binovular twins, gives some indication of the importance of genetic factors. Yet again the fact that only 40% of identical co-twins are involved, and not a figure nearer to 100%, suggests that environmental factors are probably more important in the aetiology of this condition.

Developmental Factors

It has been believed for a long time that there is an early developmental or teratological type of congenital hip displacement which is more rare than the late foetal type (Le Damany 1914); see Fig. 4.1. Putti (1929) stated that in these embryonic or foetal dislocations the femoral head developed outside the acetabular cavity. Ortolani (1948) did not believe this theory, but felt that the dislocation occurred very early in foetal life. Subsequently it has become a popular theory that there is a group of "teratological dislocations" that are associated with other congenital deformities and these are entirely different from the more common form of hip displacement.

Ruth Wynne-Davies suggested that there were two differing groups of common congenital disorders, which were separated by the fact that one of the groups appeared isolated, but the other had associated defects both in the indexed parents and the first degree relatives. In this latter group such defects occurred with greater frequency than one would find in a random sample of the population for the region.

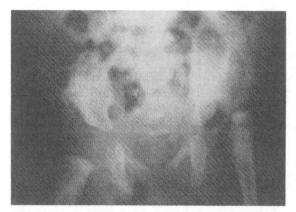

Fig. 4.1. Left CDH, "Teratological displacement". Radiologically overt and irreducible. Left CDH in an otherwise normal new-born.

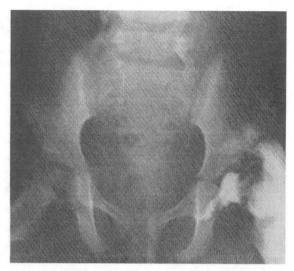

Fig. 4.2. Persistent left CDH in meningomyelocele child. The arthrogram reveals an incarcerated limbus, due to pre-natal factors, rather than post-natal muscle imbalance.

In her first group, she placed spina bifida and congenital heart disease, whereas in the second she included such conditions as idiopathic scoliosis, CDH, and talipes equino varus. These latter conditions were found to be associated with disorders that appeared to have their origin in some connective tissue defect. This, she suggested, was the developmental factor, and then chance environmental factors determined the type of congenital malformation which developed. The most obvious environmental factor in CDH is breech malposition of the foetus, but there may be other unknown factors present in first-born children that could also be significant.

Myelodysplasia

It has long been recognised that there is a high prevalence of CDH in babies born with meningomyeloceles. This is probably due to the anatomical interference with the progressive innervation of the lower limbs in the embryo, that disrupts the leg-folding mechanism and produces a greater prevalence of breech malposition in the foetus. Many such babies are born by breech presentation and have unstable hips, some of which fail to respond to neonatal splinting and develop into persistent displacements. These infants have a permanent paralysis of the gluteal muscles, causing a muscle imbalance of their hips. This is associated with an inverted limbus, as demonstrated in Fig. 4.2, the latter being produced by pre-natal displacement rather than post-natal paralysis.

Spinal dysraphism is a condition in which the conus of the spinal cord is tethered and elongated, and it is associated with a number of other anomalies affecting the cauda equina, the vertebrae,

and skin (Till 1969). Family studies have shown links between this condition and other malformations of the brain and spinal cord, such as encephalocele and spina bifida cystica (Record and McKeown 1950; Carter et al. 1968). Ruth Wynne-Davies, in 1975, related congenital scoliosis, due to multiple defects in the vertebral bodies, with classical neural tube malformations. It therefore appears that the latter (including spinal dysraphism and severe spina bifida occulta, as well as congenital scoliosis caused by multiple defects of the vertebral bodies) are all genetically and embryologically related groups of malformations (Carter et al. 1976) and occasionally may be associated with early congenital hip displacement (see Fig. 4.3).

Of more normal children born with CDH, a minority reveal stigmata of spinal dysraphism. There may be little evidence of this at birth, but occasionally unusual hair distribution, as in a fawn's tail, pigmentation of the skin, or lipomas may be seen in the lumbosacral region, as in Fig. 4.4. Later on, during the second and third years of life, the condition may become more obvious. Then their parents begin to note the persistent nocturnal enuresis and chronic constipation. At this time they begin to develop inequality of foot size and this may be associated with some persistent calcaneovalgus moulding, or the development of a mild cavus deformity of the feet. Such abnormalities are not always on the side of hip displacement. The development of the buttock muscles is often poor, but this may be partly due to the difficulties encountered in the management of CDH in these patients. Pathological

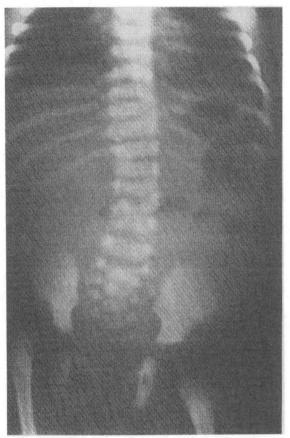

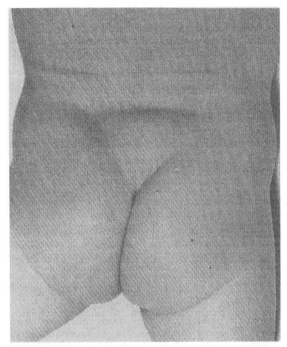

Fig. 4.4. Lumbo-sacral lipoma, spinal dysraphism. Note the unusual hair distribution and wasting of the left buttock.

Fig. 4.3. New-born with paralytic deformities of feet and right CDH. Spinal dysraphism and sphincter paralysis. Right foot calcaneo-valgus and left foot equino-varus. Note congenital scoliosis, spina bifida and obvious displacement of right hip—all genetically and embryologically related deformities.

fractures complicate their treatment and are known to have a poor prognosis. These children do not respond well to orthodox management and not infrequently there is redisplacement of the hip once the splints have been removed.

The fractures occur at the end of the long bones, especially the supracondylar area of the femur, and are similar to those in children with meningomyeloceles, indicating that there may be some common connective tissue defect in both groups of patients. Electromyographic studies of muscular development in these infants rarely show any real evidence of denervation, but the response to electrical stimulation is not normal. It has not been possible to quantify these findings to date or give them any measured prognostic significance.

Thus it appears that spinal dysraphism might have a common developmental defect with "teratological displacement" of the foetal hip joint. It might also be a developmental cause of a func-

tional delay of leg folding, later in foetal life, resulting in the more common type of CDH; and in some cases the post-natal development of increasing denervation, during infant life, appears to affect the response of such patients to orthodox management.

Sex Ratio

In 1847 Baron Dupuytren noted a female preponderance among patients with CDH, having collected 26 female cases and only three males. In most series there are five to eight girls for every boy affected: a sex ratio of between 0.2 and 0.3. This means that an incidence of 2 in 1000 total live births implies 1 in 2000 males, but 1 in 300 females.

Le Damany (1914) suggested a predisposition of girls to pre-natal dislocation, as he believed that the female sex was anthropologically higher than the males, and this meant that congenital dislocation was more frequent. He found that the female acetabulum was less oblique than that of the male. In other words it appeared more dysplastic, males having a flatter pelvis compared with the vertical form of females. He considered that CDH was the price paid for the anthropological elevation of the human species.

Subsequent anatomical research has failed to confirm any constant structural difference between the two sexes, and the more likely explanation of the sex ratio is a temporary hormonal laxity in the female foetus, lasting into the post-natal period. In the new-born it is difficult to demonstrate clinically such differences of laxity between the two sexes, but Andren (1962) claimed to be able to detect radiologically variations in the laxity of the pelvic ligaments between the two sexes. Such a temporary hormonal laxity goes a long way towards explaining the sex ratio in CDH. This form of laxity is found to be more marked during the second half of foetal life, when there is a higher production of foetal hormones, resulting from an increased stimulation provided by the maternal gonadotrophins. Hormonal joint laxity will produce a temporary instability of the foetal hip joints, making them more susceptible to mechanical environmental factors (Chapple and Davidson 1941).

Thus it appears that a genetically determined sex ratio is an important factor in the aetiology of CDH, because of its hormonal consequences.

Genetic Factors

The Herculean task of extensive family studies acceptable by modern standards has not yet been fully carried out for CDH, but it has been known for a long time that there are definite family concentrations. Muller and Seddon (1953) reported in their London series an incidence of 2.2% of sibs being affected by 1.3% of parents. Carter and Wilkinson (1964) found 5.7% of sibs to be affected, which included 4% of brothers and 7% of sisters; in this series there was a high incidence of male-indexed patients, showing a greater genetic influence than the females. In the series reported by Muller and Seddon, the incidence in the offspring was as high as that in the sibs, but in both offspring and sibs the incidence of the condition appeared to be 30 times the population incidence. This suggests that the genetic mechanism must depend on a dominant mutant gene of low manifestation rate or multifactorial inheritance, or a mixture of both. There are probably two independent mechanisms through which the genetic predisposition operates, one being the development of a shallow acetabulum, with

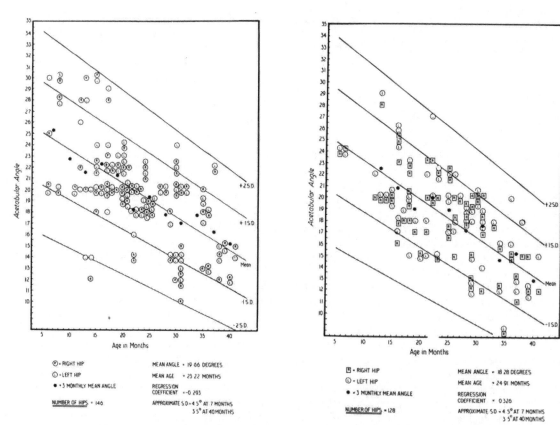

Fig. 4.5. Primary acetabular dysplasia in girls and boys (0–3 years). (Wilkinson and Carter 1960, with permission)

inadequate acetabular roof to cover fully the head of the femur (acetabular dysplasia), and the other a generalised laxity of the articular ligaments.

Primary Acetabular Dysplasia. Primary acetabular dysplasia can be measured in children over the age of 6 months and up to the age of the disappearance of the Y cartilage in the base of the acetabulum, the radiological assessment being made by Hilgenreiner's angle (1925). The normal standards of age and sex have been published (Wilkinson and Carter 1960) and it has been found that the distribution of the angle is continuous, suggesting that its genetic determination is multifactorial, as seen in the normal graphs of acetabular development in male and female children (Fig. 4.5).

When the hip has been displaced in utero, a secondary mechanical dysplasia is imposed upon the primary element, masking its true measurement, but in unilateral dislocations measurement of the non-dislocated side provides a useful guide to the probability of successful conservative treatment of the dislocation. Thus in a child with unilateral dislocation, a shallow contralateral acetabulum indicates that the end result of conservative treatment will be poor. Twenty-five per cent of cases of unilateral infantile CDH were affected and had poor results, but the response of bilateral dislocations to conservative treatment was variable (Wilkinson and Carter 1960). Thus it is believed that genetic acetabular dysplasia affects both hips equally, but its true measurement and prognostic significance can only be judged in a non-dislocated hip that has not been affected by mechanical dysplasia, as seen in Fig. 4.6.

Faber (1937) claimed to have found radiological evidence of primary acetabular dysplasia in the hips of near relatives of patients with CDH. There are difficulties in confirming his claim, as one cannot measure the acetabular angle in adult patients once the Y cartilage has disappeared, but it must be admitted that the radiographs of some parents reveal shallow acetabula with incomplete covering of the femoral head and such findings are confined to those children who exhibit primary acetabular dysplasia. It does not appear to occur in the parents of children with unilateral CDH associated with normal contralateral hip joints. Ruth Wynne-Davies (1970) carried out a radiological survey on the parents of 162 indexed patients (324 individuals), and these were compared with a control series covering the same range of patients who had radiographs taken for reasons unrelated to hip disease. She found "a shift to the left of the peak" for the parents, indicating that they had a slightly shallow acetabulum as compared with the normal public,

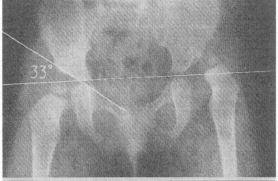
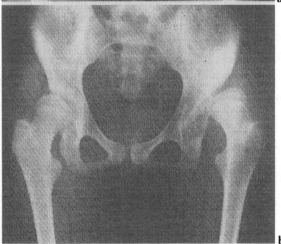

Fig. 4.6a,b. Unilateral CDH; contra-lateral normal hip dysplasia. **a** Acetabular angle of normal hip lies between 1–2 SD. **b** Ten-year follow-up after conservative treatment. (Wilkinson and Carter 1960, with permission)

but not to a significant extent. When the measurements for parents of neonatal and late-diagnosis dislocation groups were compared, there was a significant "shift to the left" of the measurements of the late-diagnosis group, but a smaller one for the neonatal group as compared with the normal controls, thus indicating that genetic acetabular dysplasia was more closely associated with the persistent congenital displacement of the hip joint in the general population.

Familial Joint Laxity. Reference has already been made to the probable importance of a temporary hormonal laxity as a factor predisposing to CDH in girls. It has been claimed that such a laxity may be extreme in affecting girls, because of the impairment of the capacity of the child's liver to destroy oestrogens (Andren and Borglin 1960).

An entirely distinct form of generalised joint laxity sometimes occurs; it is persistent and often familial, but there is no sex prevalence. Although severe forms of persistent joint laxity are often associated with Ehlers-Danlos syndrome, osteogenesis imperfecta, and Marfan's syndrome (McKusick 1956), it can also occur in isolation and be uncomplicated by other abnormalities. Some of the features are seen in Fig. 4.7. Its genetic predisposition behaves in

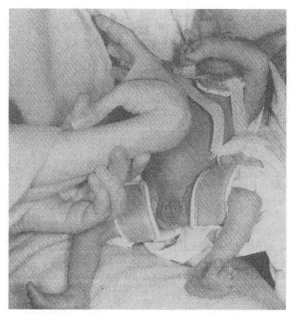

Fig. 4.8. Familial joint laxity. Mother had bilateral CDH and retains her familial joint laxity. Daughter was born with bilateral hip instability. Seen and treated at birth with Barlow splints.

families as a dominant character (Carter and Wilkinson 1964). Marked degrees of joint laxity are found in 6% of normal schoolchildren of either sex.

Using the same standards of such laxity it was found to be present in nearly three quarters of a series of boys, compared to only a third of girls with CDH. This sex prevalence is understandable, because of the alternative temporary hormonal laxity in girls. Figure 4.8 shows a mother who had bilateral CDH and has retained her familial laxity, with her first-born girl who had instability of both her hips at birth.

Pre-natal Environmental Factors

The most important pre-natal environmental factors are mechanical and appear connected with intra-uterine posture, as well as the hormonal factors previously mentioned.

The excess of breech births in patients with CDH has long been known. Muller and Seddon (1953) found in London that 16% of their series were breech born, compared with 2%–3% in the general population (1 in 40 normal births). Record and Edwards (1958) found in Birmingham a similar proportion of breech births in their series. In 174

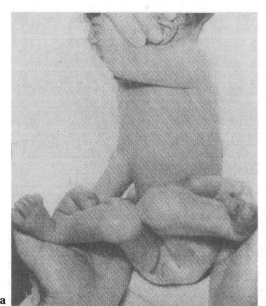

a

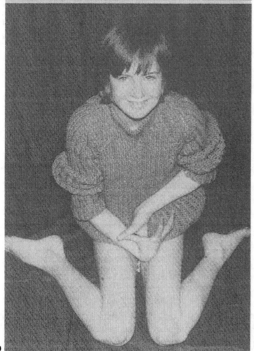

b

Fig. 4.7a,b. Familial joint laxity. **a** At birth, increased medial rotation (Wilkinson 1972, with permission). **b** Juvenile, television squat posture and thumb sign.

patients from the Hospital for Sick Children, London, Carter and Wilkinson (1964) also recorded 16% of their series to be breech born and enquiries at the respective maternity hospitals established that a further 9% had undergone therapeutic version late in pregnancy. Therefore a quarter of the patients in this series had been held in the breech malposition until late in pregnancy and there may have been others who had undergone spontaneous version. Ramsey and Macewen in an unpublished study of 25 000 new-born infants, quoted by Sherman Coleman (1978), made the following statistical observations on breech births as they relate to congenital hip disease, "1 in 35 infants will have a completely dislocated hip; 1 in 25 will have a subluxated hip and 1 in 175 will have a dislocatable hip." Thus 1 in 15 females who have had a breech birth have some degree of hip joint instability.

The excess of first-borns, 60% among patients with CDH, has also long been known, as has been the close association between being first-born and breech malposition. The breech malposition in first-borns is nearly always the frank breech posture with the hips acutely flexed and the knees extended (Vartan 1945). During her first pregnancy, the mother's abdomen and uterus have not been stretched by previous gestations and there is also a greater tendency to oligohydramnios. Both factors restrict foetal movements and seem to inferfere with leg folding. Jackson Clarke, in 1910, recognised the over-flexed position of the thighs in breech presentation as an aetiological factor, and this has also been observed by Yamamuro et al. (1977) and more recently by Tonnis (1982). Confirmation of the mechanism of intra-uterine hip displacement has been recorded in Chaps. 2 and 3, where it is shown that the combination of hormonal joint laxity and the lateral rotation breech posture of the hip leads to atraumatic displacement, with features similar to those discovered in human CDH.

Interaction of Pre-natal Factors

Although the incidence of CDH is raised in families affected by genetic acetabular dysplasia and familial joint laxity, there are many people exhibiting one of these features with stable hip joints. Yet studies of affected families, with more than one member having CDH, often reveal these two genetic features to be closely associated.

Developmental and environmental factors including acetabular dysplasia and familial joint laxity, as well as breech malposition and hormonal joint lax-

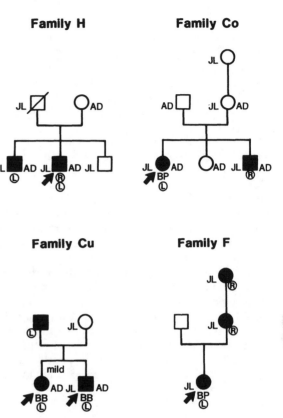

Fig. 4.9. CDH familial incidence. Four family trees illustrating the complementary effect of environmental factors upon genetic factors. (Carter and Wilkinson 1964, with permission)

ity, are not alternative, but complementary mechanisms in the production of pre-natal hip displacement. The interaction of these factors can be seen in individual families (Carter and Wilkinson 1964), as demonstrated in Fig. 4.9. Four families affected by CDH are shown. In family *H* the mother has acetabular dysplasia, but the father was dead. His wife however gave a convincing description of his previous joint laxity. This was present in three of her sons, the first-born and the second-born having CDH. These almost certainly had an acetabular dysplasia, but the third-born did not and his hips were not affected. In family *Co*, both parents had acetabular dysplasia, but only the mother and the mother's mother had joint laxity. Their first child, a girl with joint laxity and acetabular dysplasia, had a history of breech malposition. Their third child, a boy, also had joint laxity and acetabular dysplasia and both these children had CDH. Their second-born simply inherited the acetabular dysplasia, but her hips were not displaced. In family *Cu*, the mother had joint laxity and the father had a unilateral CDH.

Both children had hip displacements, the first-born being a girl did not have familial joint laxity, but had acetabular dysplasia and was breech born. The second child, a boy, had familial joint laxity and acetabular dysplasia and was also breech born. Finally in family *F* there was a marked degree of familial joint laxity associated with CDH in three successive generations.

Thus both environmental and genetic factors play a part in the causation of CDH, the former being of greater importance as they can work together, but also independently. Genetic factors usually play a secondary role, being complementary to the mechanical and hormonal factors. Perhaps the sex determination of the embryo plays the greatest part, as the sex ratio is approximately one male to seven females. Although sex determination is dependent upon genetic inheritance, its mechanism is through the production of hormonal joint laxity which is an environmental factor. In females the degree of hormonal joint laxity can be increased by a familial joint laxity, whereas in males it can be substituted by the latter and be combined with other genetic factors. Thus the environmental and genetic factors are complementary, each predisposing to the development of CDH.

Risk of CDH

Record and Edwards (1958) found that the incidence of CDH is considerably greater among sibs than among parents, and among cousins than among uncles and aunts, whereas Carter and Wilkinson (1964) found that in both offspring and sibs the incidence of the condition appears to be about 30 times the population incidence. Whereas this was once thought to be 0.7 per thousand it has now risen to 2.2 per thousand (Catford et al. 1982). These figures are based on persistent infantile dislocations in the population.

The risk of CDH to subsequent children in the family, calculated on the basis of a survey including both neonatal and late diagnosis CDH, was reported by Wynne-Davies (1970) as follows: "with normal parents the risk to subsequent sibs is 6 per cent (brothers 1 per cent and sisters 11 per cent). With an affected CDH parent, the risk for a child is 12 per cent (sons 6 per cent and daughters 17 per cent). With an affected CDH parent and one child, the risk to a second child is 36 per cent" (see Table 4.1).

Table 4.1. Risk of CDH in normal new-born (working figures) (Wilkinson and Carter 1960, Wynne-Davies 1970

General population	= 2 per 1000 live births
Boys	= 1 per 2000 live births
Girls	= 1 per 300 live births
First born girls	= 1 per 150 live births
Single breech born girls	= 1 per 15 live births

Family history of CDH

	30 × general population incidence
1 sib with CDH	= 60 per 1000
1 parent with CDH	= 120 per 1000
1 parent and child with CDH	= 360 per 1000 (nearly 1 in 3)

Post-natal Environmental Factors

The variable prevalence of CDH in different countries and races has raised the possibility of racial factors playing a part in its aetiology. It is well known that black people are almost immune to the condition (Skirving and Scadden 1979), when compared to the high susceptibility of white people and even the mongol races. In Great Britain there is a high prevalence of CDH in Wales, similar to the very high prevalence of spina bifida, which affects 8.2 per thousand live births compared with figures of 2.2 in other parts of the country. In Sweden the incidence has been estimated at 1 per thousand live births (Severin 1941), whereas in Japan the incidence is almost certainly higher than in Europe (Neel 1958), although the difference in prevalence may have disappeared in recent years. The highest incidences have been reported in Lapps (Mellbin 1962) and in certain American Indians (McDermott et al. 1960).

Nursing Habits

Lorenz in his Indian travels recorded the natural beauty of the Hindu women who never appeared to possess an ugly Trendelenburg gait, seen so frequently in Europeans. He also noted their habit of carrying the babies on their prominent hips, but was unaware of the fact that this custom might help preserve the native grace, as seen in Fig. 4.10. Cultural customs have been held responsible sometimes for raising the incidence of CDH. The Navarjo Indians in Arizona laced their infants to cradle boards with legs fully extended; this was thought to be the cause of the highest incidence of CDH in this tribe. Thus in a recent survey, 190 persons in 100 000 population were found to be affected (McDermott et al. 1960).

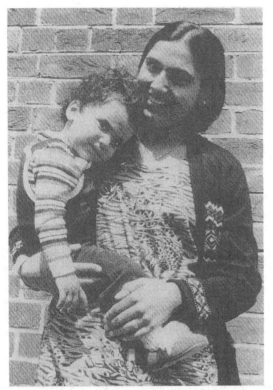

Fig. 4.10. Indian mother carrying her first-born son in traditional style, sitting him astride her hip. Unfortunately he had a persistent CDH.

According to Tonnis (1982), Buschelberger analysed the condition of the attitude of the legs when a baby was carried against the mother's body and felt that "post-natally a fetal year against the body of his mother" seemed to be necessary for the development of the acetabula, which at birth are still very immature. Yet the male child of the Indian mother in Fig. 4.10 was born with hip instability that failed to respond to his nursing care and he eventually presented with a persistent hip displacement at 18 months of age. It is also well known that Welsh mothers traditionally nurse their babies on their hips, but this has not affected the racial tendency for a high prevalence as quoted above.

Thus if post-natal nursing care has any influence as an environmental factor on the persistence of hip displacement, it must be small compared to the prenatal factors already discussed.

Seasonal Influence on Births

Record and Edwards (1958) were the first to point out that there was a high incidence of patients with persistent CDH born in the first and last quarters of the year, the summer to winter ratio being 6 to 6.6, and the males appeared to be more sensitive to the seasonal influence than females. Carter and Wilkinson (1964) confirmed this observation in infantile CDH, but later Wilkinson (1972) found a reversal of this ratio in new-born cases in which the displacement was reducible, and Ruth Wynne-Davies (1970) confirmed this finding. Most of her new-born with reducible hips were born in the summer months.

Elwood (1972) suggested that the prevalence of winter births in many congenital malformations was due to a teratogenic developmental factor that appeared to affect summer conceptions more than others. At the same time it was reported that there was a much higher prevalence of such teratogenic deformities in Great Britain than in Scandinavian countries. If we consider the summer months, when teratogenicity is higher, to be from April to September inclusively, then these patients would be born in the months January to June, which still leaves a higher percentage of summer conceptions in the persistent CDH.

Elwood's concept might well explain the absence of winter to summer ratio in the birth dates of children born with CDH in Edinburgh and in Sweden (Andren and Palmen 1963) and also the lack of sensitivity to seasonal influence in male patients. The highest incidence of babies born with CDH in Sweden is in September and November, which suggests that any summer teratogenic factor plays little part in the aetiology of this malformation in colder climates with longer winters. It might also go a long way towards explaining the greater success of neonatal diagnosis and treatment in such countries as Scotland and Sweden, as they may have fewer patients born with irreducible dislocations than regions with hotter climates such as the south of England and Wales and the Mediterranean countries.

Prevalence of CDH

When comparing the incidence of this congenital malformation reported from different centres at various times, one must remember that the earlier figures of prevalence involved only established or persistent dislocations in the population, i.e. those requiring orthopaedic care, whereas later figures were based on the prevalence of new-born with hip instability.

Perhaps the best figures for the incidence of established or persistent CDH came from England and Sweden. In a series of 50 000 children born between 1950 and 1958 in Birmingham (England) and followed up for at least 5 years, McKeown and Record (1960) reported an incidence of 0.7 per thousand, and this was accepted as the normal prevalence throughout England. A similar figure of 1 per thousand live births was reported by Severin in Sweden in 1941. Such figures can be compared with a prevalence of other skeletal congenital deformities. Spina bifida has an incidence which varies between 2.2 and 8.2 per thousand live births occurring in different regions throughout Great Britain.

Following the work of Le Damany in 1914, Putti (1929) and Ortolani (1948) described a test to detect dislocation at birth and in the neonatal period. Palmen (1961) was stimulated by this work and instigated routine examination of the hips of new-born in Sweden in 1950 and this work was followed by Von Rosen in 1962. He reported a prevalence of hip instability of 2.18 per thousand, and in 1962 Barlow increased this figure to 14.97. Mackenzie in Aberdeen undertook an extensive and enthusiastic programme of vetting of new-born during the decade 1960 to 1969 and reported in 1972 an incidence of 21.8 per thousand, which was 1 in 50 live births. All these authorities were ready to acknowledge a high level of spontaneous recovery within the first few weeks of life, in more than 50% of cases.

In Southampton the incidence of resolving and established cases between 1965 and 1978 has shown an increasing trend in each group (Catford et al. 1982). The progression from resolving to persistent or established cases has never been proved and all our attempts to eliminate resolving cases do not appear to have any influence on the incidence of established cases in the infant population. Similar findings were reported by Williamson (1972) in Northern Ireland, where it was found that the number of cases of established CDH had not fallen appreciably. In Southampton we have evidence that the incidence of CDH has been increasing since 1970; during the past 12 years there has been a threefold rise in established cases, from about 0.7 per thousand in the late 1960s to 2.2 per thousand in 1978, as seen in Fig. 4.11. The sharpest upturn in the number of established cases appeared after 1971. This has taken place in the presence of an increasing number of resolving cases, which is reflected in the figures for all cases reported during these years.

Alison MacFarlane in 1980 studied the in-patient hospital admissions of infants with CDH throughout England and Wales between 1968 and 1976 and produced similar figures to those that we have obtained in Southampton. She discovered that there was an increase in the admission of infants under 1 year of age for treatment, without any corresponding decline in the 1–4-year or the 5–9-year age group. Such figures implied either that an increas-

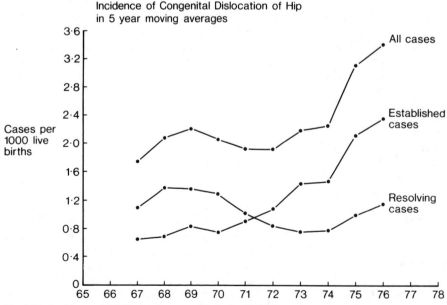

Fig. 4.11. Incidence of CDH in Southampton (Catford et al. 1982, with permission).

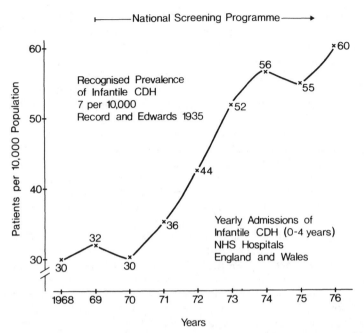

Fig. 4.12. Prevalence of CDH admitted to National Health Service hospitals in England and Wales, 1968–1976.

ing number of children were being treated for persistent dislocation of the hip, or that their treatment was involving a greater number of admissions. The latter was thought to be an unlikely cause of this increasing prevalence of admissions, as modern management tends to curtail the time spent in hospital to a minimum. The increasing prevalence of infants being admitted to National Health Service hospitals throughout England and Wales is illustrated in Fig. 4.12. Perhaps the orthodox clinical tests for hip displacement applied at birth are successful in diagnosing children with lax hip joints produced by environmental causes, but they might fail to detect those due to developmental factors. If this is so, we are diagnosing hip instability most successfully in those new-born in whom spontaneous resolution is the likely outcome. If we are to detect and treat the more difficult forms of persistent hip displacement, then it is necessary to study the aetiological factors that are responsible for their development.

Unilateral and Bilateral Hip Displacement

One of the enigmas concerning the aetiology is that there is no acceptable explanation of the distribution of hip involvement: why 75% of cases are unilateral and of these 55% are left-sided (Record and Edwards 1958). Various theories have been propounded, but

none are totally convincing. Many of the earlier workers (Bade 1900 and Ridlon 1906) went to great efforts to point out that the normal hip in unilateral cases often revealed radiological evidence of dysplasia with or without subluxation, indicating that genetic dysplasia was a prevalent factor affecting both hips. Even recently Ruth Wynne-Davies (1970) suggested that there were two groups of CDH, the first containing those with acetabular dysplasia who have a more genetic appearance affecting both hips; they also have a proportion of relatives with dislocation, the number increasing according to the severity of the degree of dysplasia. Her second group contained those cases where an environmental pre- or post-natal factor appeared more prominent, such as first-born children and also those with an excess of winter births, and these mechanical factors tended to produce a more unilateral involvement.

The mystery deepened when it was discovered that more new-born hip displacements were bilateral, as compared to the percentage of bilateral CDH in persistent cases. Ruth Wynne-Davies found that 35% of new-born hip displacements were bilateral, compared with 33% of persistent cases, but Palmen (1961) found 47.3% to be bilateral in the new-born. MacKenzie (1972) discovered that bilateral involvement was more common than unilateral at birth, but when one side was involved it was more often the left than the right. His figures showed a ratio of 19:35 for right to left hip involvement at birth, but the spontaneous cure rate was higher on the left than the right, and by 3 weeks the ratio of instability was 47:56. He found that for some reason persistent displacement requiring operative treatment occurred more commonly on the left side, the ratio being 19:40. Thus there appeared to be pre-natal and post-natal mechanical factors increasing the prevalence and persistency of hip displacement on the left side.

Dunn (1976) expressed the most popular Hippocratic theory that the prevalence of left hip displacement was due to malposition in utero. He found the left hip was displaced twice as often as the right at birth, and he claimed that this was due to the foetus tending to lie with its back on the left side of the uterus twice as commonly as it did on the right. Taylor (1976) suggested that a cause for intra-uterine asymmetry could be the torsion of the uterus to the right (in most pregnancies), which causes the bladder to be displaced to the right. This displacement leaves more room on the left for the left occiput position of the foetal head when it is anterior or transverse. Dunn (1976) believed that the leg of the foetus lying posteriorly was much more likely to be dislocated than that lying anteriorly: "because the mother's spine juts out into the abdominal cavity, the leg lying posteriorly is more likely to be adducted and hence to lie in the position in which the hip joint is more vulnerable to dislocation". There are two objections to this theory. The first is the evidence recorded in Chaps. 1–3 which indicates that lateral rotation is more important than adduction in the intra-uterine dislocating mechanism. The second is that 50% of new-born with CDH have been in the breech malposition during the critical time of their intra-uterine existence, i.e. within the last 3 months of pregnancy. This would indicate that the right hip is exposed to such intra-uterine mechanical factors as described by Dunn, rather than the left hip which is more frequently affected. Perhaps this explains MacKenzie's reference (1972) to Frew's observation, "that CDH was unrelated to the side nearest the maternal spine".

More recent evidence concerning the position of the foetus in utero indicates that the lie is longitudinal in 99% of cases, being cephalic presentation in 95% and breech presentation in 4%. In the cephalic posture 75% lie laterally, 35% being on the right and 40% on the left. In the breech presentation, the left sacro-anterior lie is the most common, as demonstrated in Fig. 4.13. According to Dunn's theory this would expose the right hip to a greater mechanical embarrassment than the left, and it is still necessary to explain bilateral hip displacement.

Thus it appears that there are many unexplained factors in the extrinsic intra-uterine environmental theories concerning the selection of intra-uterine posture and the aetiology of breech malposition and pre-natal hip displacement; and so it is necessary to look at intrinsic factors in the developing foetus which might be common to all these problems. Sir Denis Browne (1936) in his paper on congenital deformities of mechanical origin stated that the notion that they may be caused by pressure in utero dated back at least to Hippocrates. He felt that "to prove the question one way or another by direct observation is at present impossible and it appears ever likely to remain so". Consequently he was reduced to a method of comparing what abstract argument showed to be the consequence of the granting of a hypothesis under test, with that which was actually found in real life: "If the results of such abstract inductive reasoning of this sort coincided with the observations over a wide and complicated range, the truth of the hypothesis on which the reasoning was conducted is proved as nearly absolutely as most things can be in this world." On such grounds a hypothesis is proposed, that the prevalence of left foetal intra-uterine position is due to the intrinsic factor of cerebral dominance through its influence on the progressive innervation of the embryonic and foetal limbs. What evidence have we to support such a hypothesis, which might explain the prevalence of intra-uterine hip displacement, and also the post-natal persistence of left hip displacement as compared to bilateral and right hip involvement?

Firstly the watertight clinical evidence gained from the examination of new-born revealing all the features of pre-natal influence without any post-natal distortion. Such evidence involves plagiocephaly, torticollis, scoliosis, hip displacement, and moulding deformities of the feet. All these features are wrapped up in one condition, namely the "moulded baby syndrome" described by Denis Browne (1965) as well as Lloyd-Roberts and Pilcher (1965). They described an intra-uterine moulding of the new-born, more commonly seen in boys, in which there was a flattening of the left side of the head associated with a right torticollis and a left scoliosis, with a pelvic tilt to the left and limited abduction of the left hip, as seen in Fig. 4.13. More recently Goode and Walker (1983) described the same moulded baby syndrome and unilateral tight hip with all the same features, with pelvic obliquity resulting in a unilateral loss of hip abduction in flexion which may be confused with congenital dislocation or dysplasia of the hip. They discovered that there was a flattening of the front of the forehead on the same side as the affected hip, which they

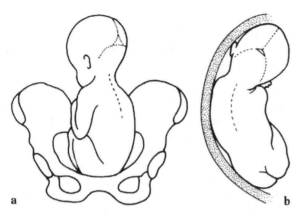

Fig. 4.13a,b. Intra-uterine posture and its effect. **a** The left sacro-anterior lie, commonest breech posture. **b** The moulding of the uterine wall to produce plagiocephaly, torticollis, scoliosis, and pelvic tilt.

called plagiocephaly. This coincided with the observations made in a review of all new-born in Southampton (Wilkinson 1972). Ruth Wynne-Davies (1968), when studying familial idiopathic scoliosis, found that plagiocephaly was a transient deformity associated with infantile scoliosis and in all cases the plagiocephaly agreed with the side of the curve. In other words, 88% of infants had left-sided curves and the left side of the head appeared flattened anteriorly. She found in her control group that 11% of the normal population had such plagiocephaly, but this was distributed equally between the left and right sides. Thus it appears that there is a mechanical factor in infantile scoliosis which tends to act pre-natally, producing plagiocephaly and scoliosis on the ipsilateral side.

Professor J. I. P. James's paper on the aetiology of scoliosis (1970) suggested that a posterolateral plagiocephaly came on within a few days or weeks after birth, and he quoted Hay who thought that the plagiocephaly probably arose through the baby lying in an oblique position with the still plastic skull flowing into the shape. Such a result of gravity acting on the skull could point to a similar effect of gravity on the infant's spine. Thus he implied that post-natal posterior plagiocephaly was due to the nursing of the new-born infant and depended on the mother's decision to nurse her baby on its left or right side. It appears that this choice, however, coincided with the pre-natal position in utero, as it resulted in a left scoliosis in both cases.

A large amount of research has gone on in recent years on head orientation pre-natally, during birth and in the neonatal period and its association with hand preference in the first year of life (Goodwin and Mitchell 1981). Without going into great detail,

there is convincing evidence that 59% of neonates prefer to lie with their heads turning to the right, 45% exhibiting a consistent right preference. It has also been noted that the pre-natal preference of left intra-uterine position is always linked to a post-natal right-handed preference, whereas the relationship between right intra-uterine position to left-handedness is not so clear-cut. Smart et al. (1980) discarded the hypothesis of Bakan et al. (1973) that handedness was associated with birth stress and trauma. They also found that there was no clear-cut evidence of left-handed throwers having any association with birth order. Foetal position has also been associated with later hand preference by Koppel (1971), Watson (1924), and Churchill et al. (1962), but it was not clear whether the foetal posture dictated both. Previously it has been thought that cerebral dominance had a genetic origin, whereas Melekian (1981) stated that anatomical findings showing hemispheric asymmetry in some areas of the brain in neonates make the existence of a corresponding functional asymmetry at birth very likely. From all this information one might feel that intra-uterine position is in some way dependent upon the development of embryological or foetal cerebral dominance.

When we came to assess such factors in our CDH patients, it was necessary at first to obtain normal controls. In normal schoolchildren we found that 12% of boys and 9% of girls either wrote or threw a ball with their left hand and this was determined in a survey of 333 normal children. With regard to our patients with persistent hip displacement, 13% of left CDH, compared with 20% of right CDH and 23% of bilateral CDH, are left-handed. In bilateral cases 6 out of 14 boys (nearly 50%) were left-handed, whereas 2 out of 21 girls (less than 10%) were similarly affected. Thus there seems to be no increase in left cerebral dominance in left CDH, but there is a definite increase in right-sided CDH and bilateral cases. A similar survey is now being carried out in new-born cases.

It thus appears that CDH might well eventually turn out to be similar to pes cavus, in that the percentage of idiopathic cases becomes gradually reduced with the recognition of developmental neurogenic disorders and genetically determined connective tissue disorders (Brewerton et al. 1962).

The relationship between cerebral dominance, head orientation, hand preference and post-natal nursing factors influencing the persistence of hip instability is far more obvious. It is known that if a mother places her child on its dominant side and restricts the dominant upper limb, the child will become restless and cry. This means that the mother will be influenced to nurse her child on its non-dominant side, if she has not been persuaded to nurse in the prone position. Such a nursing influence will not only aggravate any pre-natal plagiocephaly and tendency to scoliosis, but it will also impose extension and adduction upon the non-dominant hip, which is more likely to be on the left side, as the majority of new-born have a right-handed preference. This could well account for MacKenzie's observation (1972) that persistent displacement requiring operative treatment occurred more commonly on the left side.

Factors Involved in the Increasing Prevalence of CDH

A study of known aetiological factors, including a family history of CDH, sex ratio, first-born and breech delivery rates, birth weight, maternal age, and familial joint laxity, has revealed no increasing trend in any of these factors which might account for the gradual rise in the prevalence of CDH. Amniocentesis for the diagnosis of foetal abnormality was thought to be a cause of orthopaedic abnormalities, due to the effect of a sudden withdrawal of a volume of amniotic fluid on joint development (Medical Research Council Working Party 1979); but as only one of the mothers in our series has been subjected to this, it has been discounted as a practical factor in our series. Maternal smoking habits were reported to be a possible cause of increasing prevalence of orthopaedic deformities (Noble et al. 1978), but an equal number of our mothers were non-smokers to those who had persisted with the habit, and there was no difference found between those mothers who had admitted to smoking during pregnancy and subsequently having a child with CDH, as compared with a group of matching controls.

Perinatal mortality has dropped in the Southampton district from 20.8 per thousand in 1970 to 11.3 per thousand in 1976, as reported by Jones and Radford in 1978. This was considered to be a possible factor, as an increased perinatal mortality had been reported in malformed children with CDH by Dunn (1976). Yet even if all the babies with CDH survived in the 1970s which might have died in the 1960s, the dramatic increase in the incidence of the deformity could not be sufficiently explained by a declining stillbirth rate.

The only major impact on the birth rate in the past 10 years has been the increasing popularity of the hormonal birth-control pill. This was introduced in the late 1960s, but did not become popular until 1970, which coincides with the increase in the prevalence of CDH. The birth pill originally contained more oestrone than progesterone, but because of thrombotic complications the ratio has been reversed. It is difficult to explain how the use of the birth-control pill preceding the affected pregnancy could influence either the maternal or foetal hormonal *milieu intérieur* during the last 3 months of pregnancy, even had the mother persisted with her programme during the first few months. It is known that the pregnancy hormones have a tendency to depress pituitary function and there is a possibility that the birth-control pill may produce a "whiplash of hyperactivity" after its discontinuation. This could be responsible for the stimulation of the foetal adrenal glands and even the placenta during the pregnancy. Such could account for an increase in the hormonal factor. Although there is a possibility that the birth pill does have some effect upon the foetal blood levels in subsequent pregnancies, there is as yet no information in the literature concerning any teratogenesis with oestrone or progesterone and none indicating that the foetal levels of oestrone and progesterone are otherwise affected.

Thus the incidence of CDH is increasing, but there is no evidence to explain why this is taking place. Similar rises have been reported from Israel (Khingberg et al. 1976) and the United States (Center for Disease Control 1975, Congenital Malformations Surveillance Report). Such a general increase through the western world would suggest an environmental factor as a cause, but as yet we have been unable to identify one with certainty. It is interesting to note, however, that in Japan, where the birth-control pill is not popular, there is no evidence of any increasing prevalence of CDH, as reported by Yamamuro in a personal communication (1983).

Summary

1) The aetiology of this common congenital deformation is multifactorial, involving developmental and environmental factors.

2) Racial prevalence is variable and this may be due to either pre-natal developmental factors or post-natal environmental influences, resulting in an increase in Celtic races, but providing an immunity in Indian and African people.

3) Familial factors appear to be genetic and are responsible for family histories of CDH. They are either recessive, as in genetic acetabular dysplasia, or dominant, as seen in familial joint laxity.

4) Stigmata of spinal dysraphism can be recognised in otherwise apparently normal children with CDH. Rarely this condition is associated with early foetal hip displacement, but more commonly it is seen in those with late foetal displacement, and only becomes apparent post-natally when it affects normal growth and muscular development.

5) The majority of children with CDH reveal no evidence of developmental factors and their condition must therefore be considered idiopathic in origin. As with pes cavus, the percentage of otherwise normal children may dwindle in the future, as we come to recognise other cryptic aetiological factors.

6) Environmental factors appear to be far more important than developmental tendencies, especially the pre-natal hormonal joint laxity and breech malposition. These factors appear to be effective in isolation, but become more productive when interacting with developmental factors.

7) The prevalence of early and persistent cases of CDH has more than doubled in the past 12 years, but the main reason for this increase has not yet been confirmed.

References

Andren L (1962) Pelvic instability in newborns. Acta Radiol [Suppl] 212

Andren L, Borglin N (1960) A disorder of oestrogen metabolism as a causal factor of congenital dislocation of the hip. Acta Orthop Scand 30:169

Andren L, Palmen K (1963) Seasonal variation in birth dates of infants with congenital dislocation of the hip. Acta Orthop Scand 33(2):127

Bade P (1900) quoted by Vernon L. Hart (1948) Congenital dysplasia of the hip joint and sequelae. Charles E. Thomas, Illinois

Bakan P, Dibb G, Reed P (1973) Handedness and birth stress. Neuropsychologia 11:363–366

Barlow TG (1962) Early diagnosis and treatment of congenital dislocation of the hip joint. J Bone Joint Surg 44B:292

Brewerton D, Sandifer P, Sweetnam R (1962) Pes cavus. British Orthopaedic Spring Meeting. J Bone Joint Surg 44B(3)

Browne D (1936) Congenital deformities of mechanical origin. Proc R Soc Med 29:1409

Browne D (1965) Congenital postural scoliosis. Br Med J 2:565

Carter CO (1962) Human heredity. Pelican Books A523. Penguin Books, Harmondsworth, Middlesex, England

Carter CO, Wilkinson JA (1964) Genetic and environmental factors in the aetiology of congenital dislocation of the hip. Clin Orthop 33:119

Carter C, David P, Laurence K (1968) A family study of major central nervous system malformation in South Wales. J Med Genet 5:81–106

Carter C, Evans K, Till K (1976) Spinal dysraphism: Genetic relation to neural tube malformations. J Med Genet 13:343–350

Catford JC, Bennet GC, Wilkinson JA (1982) Congenital hip dislocation: an increasing and still uncontrolled disability. Br Med J 285:1527

Center for Disease Control (1975) Congenital malformations surveillance report. Center for Disease Control, Atlanta, Georgia

Chapple C, Davidson T (1941) A study of the relationship between foetal position and certain congenital deformities. J Paediatr 18:483

Churchill J, Igna E, Senf R (1962) The association of position at birth and handedness. Pediatrics 29:307–309

Clarke JJ (1910) Congenital dislocation of the hip. Ballière, Tindall & Cox, London

Coleman S (1978) Congenital dysplasia and dislocation of the hip. Mosby, St. Louis

Dunn P (1976) Perinatal observations on the aetiology of congenital dislocation of the hip. Clin Orthop 119:11

Dupuytren G (1847) Injuries and diseases of bones. Translated by F. Le Gros Clark for the Sydenham Society, London

Elwood JH (1972) Quoted in Editorial, Lancet 2:195

Faber A (1937) Erbbiologische Untersuchungen über die Anlage zur "angeborenen" Huftverrenkung. Z Orthop 66:140

Goode C, Walker G (1983) Moulded baby syndrome and unilateral "tight" hips. Br Med J 287:1675

Goodwin R, Mitchell G (1981) Head orientation position during birth and in infant neonatal period and hand preference at 19 weeks. Child dev 52: 819–826

Hilgenreiner H (1925) On the early diagnosis and treatment of congenital dislocation of the hip. Med Klin 21(1):385

Idelberger K (1951) The genetic pathology of so-called congenital dislocation of the hip. Urban & Schwarzenberg, Munich

James JIP (1970) The aetiology of scoliosis. J Bone Joint Surg 52B(3):410

Jones C, Radford M (1978) Perinatal morbidity and one-year infant morbidity. Br Med J 1:325

Khingberg MA, Chen R, Chemke J, Levin S (1976) Rising rates of congenital dislocation of the hip. Lancet 1:298

Koppel H (1971) Letter to the Editor of Scientific American 224:9

Le Damany P (1914) Congenital luxation of the hip. Am J Orthop Surg 11(4):541

Lloyd-Roberts GC, Pilcher MF (1965) Structural idiopathic scoliosis in infancy. A study of the natural history of 100 patients. J Bone Joint Surg 47B:520

MacFarlane A (1980) Congenital dislocation of the hip—an epidemiological conundrum. J Mat Child Health. January, 1980, p 13

MacKenzie I (1972) Congenital dislocation of the hip: the development of a regional service. J Bone Joint Surg 54B:18

McDermott W, Deuschle K, Adair J, Fulmer H, Laughlin B (1960) Introducing modern medicine in a Navajo community. Science 131:197

McKeown T, Record RG (1960) Congenital malformations. Ciba Foundation Symposium. Churchill, London

McKusick VA (1956) Heritable disorders of connective tissue. Mosby, St. Louis

Medical Research Council Working Party (1978) An assessment of the hazards of amniocentesis. Br J Obstet Gynaecol, London

Noble T, Pullen C, Craft A, Leonard M (1978) Difficulties in diagnosing and managing congenital dislocation of the hip. Br Med J 2:620–623

Ortolani M (1948) La lussazione congenita dell'anca: Nuovi criteri diagnostici e profilattico-correttivi. Cappelli, Bologna

Palmen K (1961) Preluxation of the hip joint. Acta Paediatr 50: Supplement 129

Putti V (1929) Early treatment of congenital dislocation of the hip. J Bone Joint Surg 11:798–809

Record R, McKeown T (1950) Congenital malformations of the

central nervous system. Risks of malformation in sibs of malformed individuals. Br J Prev Soc Med 4:217–220

Record RG, Edwards JH (1958) Environmental influences related to the aetiology of congenital dislocation of the hip. Br J Prev Soc Med 12(1):8–22

Ridlon J (1906) Spontaneous dislocation at the hip joint. Surg Gynecol Obstet 2:613–617

Severin E (1941) Contribution to the knowledge of congenital dislocation of the hip joint. Acta Chir Scand 84:Supplement 63

Skirving A, Scadden W (1979) The African neonatal hip and its immunity from congenital dislocation. J Bone Joint Surg 61B:339–341

Smart J, Jeffrey C, Richards B (1980) A retrospective study of the relationship between birth history and handedness at 6 years. Early human development, vol 4, no 1, pp 79–88. Elsevier North-Holland Biomedical, Amsterdam

Taylor ES (1976) Beck's obstetrical practise and fetal medicine, 10th edn. William & Wilkins, Baltimore

Till K (1969) Spinal dysraphism: a study of congenital malformations of the back. Dev Med Child Neurol 10:471–478

Tonnis D (1982) Congenital hip dislocation—Avascular necrosis. Thieme-Stratton, New York Stuttgart

Vartan CK (1945) The behaviour of the foetus in utero with special reference to the incidence of breech presentation at term. J Obstet Gynaecol 52:417

Von Rosen S (1962) Diagnosis and treatment of congenital dislocation of the hip joint in the newborn. J Bone Joint Surg 44B:284

Watson J (1924) Behaviourism. University of Chicago Press, Chicago

Wilkinson JA (1972) A post-natal survey for congenital dislocation of the hip. J Bone Joint Surg 54B:40–49

Wilkinson JA, Carter CO (1960) Congenital dislocation of the hip. The results of conservative treatment. J Bone Joint Surg 42B(4):669–688

Williamson J (1972) Difficulties of early diagnosis and treatment of congenital dislocation of the hip in Northern Ireland. J Bone Joint Surg 54B(1):13

Wynne-Davies R (1968) Familial idiopathic scoliosis. J Bone Joint Surg 50B(1):24

Wynne-Davies R (1970) A family study of neonatal and late diagnosis congenital dislocation of the hip. J Med Genet 7:315

Wynne-Davies R (1975) Congenital vertebral anomalies: Aetiology and relationship to spina bifida cystica. J Med Genet 12:136–145

Yamamuro T, Hama H, Takeda T, Shikata J, Sanada H (1977) Biomechanical and hormonal factors in the etiology of congenital dislocation of the hip joint. Int Orthop (SICOT) 1:231–236

5 CDH at Birth and in the First Ten Months of Life: Its Diagnosis and Management

> A simple clinical method, easily learned and quickly applied, adding less than a minute to the time of the examination to which every new born child is entitled, could be used to take the sting out of congenital dislocation of the hip as a crippling disorder.
>
> *H. J. Seddon* (1962)

Although more than two thousand years have passed since Hippocrates (460–370 B.C.) identified that "those persons, then, are most maimed who have experienced the dislocation in utero", there is still no consensus of orthopaedic opinion on the advent of hip displacement. Is it a pre-natal congenital deformation present in varying degrees at birth, or is it entirely a post-natal acquired deformity?

Putti (1929) and Ortolani (1948) were the first to suggest a pre-natal subluxation, present at birth, which either recovered spontaneously or went on to develop into a permanent luxation. Hart (1948) and Beckett Howarth (1963) believed that affected new-born had simply a dysplasia or laxity of ligaments at birth and called the term congenital dislocation a misnomer.

Even today the controversy persists and the relative failure to diagnose 30%–50% of persistent cases at birth has led some to suggest that they are a late post-natal event (MacKenzie 1972), and this would account for patients who appear for the first time months after the most stringent vetting.

History of Early Diagnosis

For many centuries the habit of examining new-born hips for instability was practised by mothers on their daughters throughout Central Europe, France, and Italy and when instability was discovered the children were nursed with pillows between their legs. This was an attempt to stabilise the hip joints, more for cosmetic than functional reasons. It is therefore surprising that medical interest in this practice was not reported before 1864, when Roser recorded that some new-born had loose hip joints, which could be luxated by adducting the thighs and then reduced by abduction. He ended his observations with the words "I believe that many of these cases, indeed most of them, would be curable if the deformities were discovered in the new-born and then the abduction bandages were immediately applied." He declared that his report had remained dormant for 15 years before he wrote it, but even then his ideas appeared to be ignored by the contemporary orthopaedic schools.

No systematic investigation of new-born with hip instability was undertaken until the work of Le Damany in 1914. After extensive research he came to the conclusion that there were two separate groups of hip displacement, including a rare teratological luxation developing in early foetal life and a more common anthropologic luxation occurring later. This latter group could be detected, because of the instability of the hip joint, soon after birth.

Le Damany's Test for Hip Instability

This appears to have been a unilateral test, checking one hip at a time by stabilising the pelvis with one hand and examining the opposite hip with the other. The joint was dislocated gently by displacing the femoral head, using the thumb to apply firm pressure on the medial aspect of the thigh, and then lifting the femoral head in and out of the acetabulum by applying pressure with the middle finger over the greater trochanter. This manoeuvre lifted the femoral head into the acetabulum and the withdrawal of pressure allowed it to slip out again. Le Damany recognised the likelihood of spontaneous recovery in these cases, but he also devised a splint to maintain reduction in order to expedite the cure. Yet he was far from convinced that this group of unstable hips at birth was a potential source of persistent dislocation beyond infant life!

The orthopaedic world was again stirred when Putti (1934) in Italy discovered that all cases of congenital hip preluxation could be diagnosed radiologically during the first year of life, and he advised that treatment should start immediately the diagnosis was made. More than 95% of his cases were treated successfully by splinting the child's legs in abduction, but a minority persisted as permanent hip displacements! This work stimulated Ortolani to undertake anatomical and clinical surveys, and in 1948 he wrote his monumental paper on "La Lussazione Congenita Dell'Anca". This outstanding contribution has never been published in English, but the author was fortunate enough to be given a personal translation of the manuscript by Dr Ponsetti, in Iowa. Ortolani came to the conclusion that the clinical diagnosis was far more critical than radiological examination, including arthrography of the hip. He described his "signs of probability of dislocation", paying heed to many external features, including the lateral rotation of the lower extremity in the position of abandonment, as well as describing the sign of *scatto* or "snapping sign".

The Ortolani Sign of Hip Instability

To demonstrate this sign, the patients were placed in a supine position with the thighs flexed and at right angles to the pelvis, both knees being slightly inwardly rotated. A movement of abduction and lateral rotation of both thighs was produced by holding the knees in the palms of the hands, with the thumbs on the inner aspects and the fingers over the outer aspect of the thighs. The thumbs applied pressure in a lateral direction, whereas the fingers exerted a similar pressure over the greater trochanters in a medial direction. The former displaced the femoral head over the posterior rim of the acetabulum, whereas the latter reduced the femoral heads producing the sensation of jumping in and out of the sockets. Ortolani noted that the persistency of this snapping sign during the period of treatment was of poor prognosis, indicating that hip instability might not respond to abduction splints and sometimes persist as permanent displacement.

Palmen was so inspired by this work that in 1950 he took Ortolani's methods to his native Sweden and began to practise early diagnosis of CDH there. In 1961 he published the early results in a monograph recording his experiences. He used the same diagnostic technique of bilateral examination as developed by Ortolani, and confirmed that the clinical findings were far more dependable than any radiological tests in early post-natal life.

Palmen's Provocative Test of Hip Instability

A technique was developed in which instability was provoked by forced subluxation of the hip joint, using one hand to fix the pelvis and testing the opposite hip with the other hand, simulating the manoeuvre previously described by Le Damany. He found that the provocative test was often positive when the original Ortolani test was negative, but such cases usually underwent spontaneous recovery and he was not certain as to the significance of his own test; 47.3% of his cases were bilateral at birth and the remainder were unilateral preluxations. The overall prevalence was approximately 5.7 per thousand new-born, compared to the 0.9 per thousand which was the prevalence of persistent dislocations, previously reported by Severin in the same area in 1946. Palmen recognised that complete luxation of the hip could occur before birth and in these cases his sign might be negative; but the condition should be suspected when there was limited abduction of the hip joint at birth!

This work spread rapidly to other parts of Sweden and Von Rosen recorded his experiences in 1962. He was the first to declare that all congenital dislocations presented as unstable hips at birth, believing that total displacement and irreducibility were postnatal developments. Thus he believed that every case should be diagnosed within the first few days of life by the snapping sign. Barlow introduced the work of Von Rosen into Britain in 1957. He used the modified Ortolani test, similar to that described by Le Damany and also by Palmen as his provocative test. It involved a unilateral examination, using the opposite hand to fix the pelvis in order to manipulate the suspected hip joint. Barlow agreed with Von Rosen that all cases could be diagnosed within the first few days of life and that any impediment to reduction was due to post-natal contractures.

The subsequent diligent search for CDH at birth has not been so successful as promised by earlier workers. Even in the most dedicated of paediatric centres throughout Great Britain, the exhaustive efforts have failed to reduce the number of persistent cases to any appreciable degree. When our present figures are compared with the prevalence reported in Great Britain by Record and Edwards in 1958, before neonatal diagnosis was practised, there is no evidence of any decrease in the number of persistent cases as a result of all our efforts. In 1968 Robert Owen stated, "we suspect that in spite of constant vigilance and routine testing by means of the Ortolani sign and its variants, even the expert may sometimes fail", and in the same volume of the Journal of Bone and Joint Surgery (54B, 1972), his words were re-echoed by Mitchell, Williamson, MacKenzie, and Wilkinson. David Jones (1977) recorded similar feelings when he stated, "notwithstanding the major pioneer work of Von Rosen and Barlow, it is apparent from this study that neonatal examinations at birth will not eliminate the problem of congenital dislocation of the hip".

Post-natal Presentation

The development of untreated congenital hip displacement, from birth to skeletal maturity, can be conveniently divided into four stages. Clear definition of these groups will exclude confusion and lead to meaningful discussion. Although such divisions are artificial and overlap one another, they are based on post-natal anatomical development and prove useful when laying down the guidelines for future management.

New-born CDH (0–4 weeks)

At birth, the new-born reveals all the features of pre-natal influence, without any post-natal distortion. There has been no time to affect the clinical evidence, nor influence the response to treatment. Opinions vary as to when post-natal factors begin to influence the pre-natal deformation of the hip joint. Von Rosen (1962) and Fredensborg (1977)

believed that such changes begin to develop within the first few days of life, but MacKenzie (1972) found that there was little or no difference in the response of CDH to treatment within the first 3 weeks of life, indicating that little change had developed during this time. After the first month, however, the response to treatment decreases owing to the development of contractures of the capsule of the hip joint and the adductor muscles. Secondary bony deformation is also caused by persistent post-natal posture.

Radiology at this stage is confusing and is not very helpful to diagnosis.

Neonatal CDH (1–10 months)

During this phase, the clinical diagnosis can become more obvious in the minority of persistent cases, because of the development of post-natal contractures. Yet the diagnosis becomes more obscure in the majority of cases that are recovering spontaneously.

The radiological features remain confusing until the appearance of the proximal epiphysis, but this can sometimes be delayed in abnormal hips until after the tenth month.

Infantile CDH (10 months–3 years)

In these cases of persistent hip displacement, the clinical signs become more obvious as the child grows older and begins to stand and walk. Hip displacement is more evident in unilateral cases, where there is a normal leg for comparison, and this means that diagnosis is made sooner than in bilateral cases.

The division of the 10-month neonate from the infantile group is dependent upon the radiological appearance of the proximal femoral epiphyses. This not only makes the radiological diagnosis obvious, but the appearance of the ossific centre heralds the establishment of a mature blood supply. It also strengthens the femoral head to resist mechanical compression (see Chap. 3). Thus the radiological appearance of the proximal femoral epiphysis lowers the prevalence of epiphysitis, which is the commonest iatrogenic complication of management.

Juvenile CDH (from 3 years to skeletal maturity)

When the infant has reached the end of the third year of post-natal development, the growth of the femur is greater than that of the adductor and hamstring muscles. The degree of femoral head displacement is also aggravated by the increasing weight of the child and the longer hours of standing and walking. Deformation of the capsule and other soft tissues continues to develop. All these factors make the reduction of persistent displacement far more difficult. Surgery is required and it is often necessary to undertake more extensive measures than those necessary in infantile cases.

Congenital Displacement at Birth

Although the expert orthopaedic surgeon should be able to diagnose all degrees of CDH at birth, the early diagnosis is not as simple as suggested by Von Rosen and Barlow. The detection of hip instability is dependent upon a high standard of training, involving dedicated doctors and nurses. There is an art or an authority which must be cultivated in order to soothe and relax the child, to provide the necessary conditions to be able to undertake such critical assessment successfully. This cannot be accomplished on a child who is kicking and struggling against non-maternal intrusion. It must also be accepted that there are some experienced members of the medical and nursing profession who are incapable of developing the techniques of neonatal examination!

The dependence upon one clinical sign, that of hip instability, and the failure to recognise the fact that the Ortolani sign may be negative in children with complete hip displacement, leads to a high proportion of missed cases, as proved in retrospective studies. If greater success is to be obtained in the diagnosis of this most common congenital deformation of the skeletal system at birth, it is necessary to recognise all the signs of breech malposition as well as those of hip displacement. "We must learn to examine the attitude of the entire foetus in our routine examination of the new born infant, so that certain obscure deformities not apparent on ordinary inspection may be detected" (Chapple and Davidson 1941). Ortolani did not depend upon the orthodox tests for hip instability, but described twelve signs of "probability of hip dislocation" in the new-born, the last being the sign of *scatto*.

Signs of Breech Malposition

If it is accepted that this is the commonest form of mechanical embarrassment to the intra-uterine

development of the foetal hip joint, it must be recognised that it may be adopted for a temporary phase in the leg-folding mechanism, or it may persist throughout much of foetal development. Thus the overt evidence of breech malposition may be seen in varying degrees in the new-born (Wilkinson 1972). Some of the signs are present in those eventually born by cephalic delivery, but they are more obvious in those that have been subjected to persistent breech malposition, and appear to be even more evident in those with congenital hip displacement. It is therefore necessary to recognise each sign in the new-born population, in order to attract one's attention to the hip joints. If there is any doubt about diagnosis, such new-born should be followed up until one is certain that the hips are clinically or even radiologically normal.

Pre-natal Moulding. Chapple and Davidson were the first to refer to the birth posture as the "position of comfort", for when the new-born is wrapped in this position it relaxes and tends to fall asleep, as before birth it was used to this cramped position (Fig. 5.1).

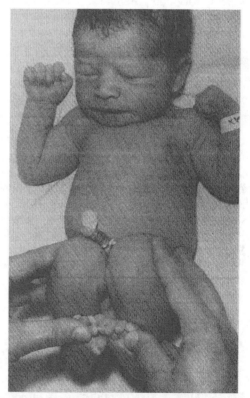

Fig. 5.1. The position of comfort, full flexion, cephalic presentation. Note that the newborn falls asleep when placed in its birth posture, which represents the pre-natal posture. (Wilkinson 1972, with permission)

Normally the evidence of such intra-uterine moulding disappears within the first few days of life, but in new-born that have been previously subjected to prolonged breech malposition the signs may persist during the first 4 weeks of life. It is believed that such pre-natal moulding is due to mechanical restriction, imposed upon a foetus with increased compressibility, due to excessive soft tissue laxity (Fig. 5.2). A survey performed in Southampton (Wilkinson 1972) revealed that the birth postures became increasingly apparent, being least evident in cephalic (vertex) deliveries compared to breech born, but being even more overt in new-born with CDH, especially when there is a negative Ortolani test. In the latter, there is a marked limitation of abduction of the affected hip joint at birth, proving it to be a pre-natal and not a post-natal feature. The various patterns of posture are recorded in Fig. 5.3.

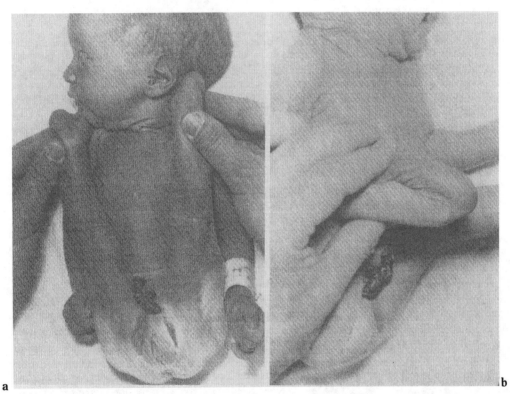

a   b

Fig. 5.2a,b. Pre-natal moulding, hyperextended breech malposition. Note that the babe is relaxed and there is excessive dorsiflexion of the foot due to familial joint laxity.

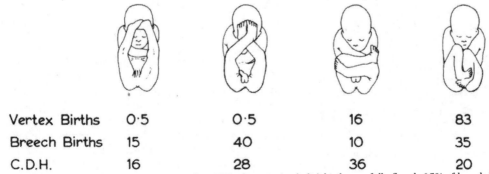

Vertex Births	0·5	0·5	16	83
Breech Births	15	40	10	35
C.D.H.	16	28	36	20

Fig. 5.3. Patterns of birth posture. Note that 83% of vertex (cephalic) births are fully flexed. 65% of breech births have delayed leg-folding. 80% of new-born CDH reveal evidence of breech malposition. (Wilkinson 1972, with permission)

It can be seen that there is little evidence of interference with the leg-folding mechanism in the cephalic or vertex deliveries, whereas more than half of the cases of breech birth had delayed leg-folding, and 80% of those with CDH were likewise affected. The new-born posture identified in nearly every case with CDH is shown in Fig. 5.4. This became recognised as "the position of dislocation" and it could only be imposed on new-born with an excessive range of lateral rotation of the flexed thighs. This is in keeping with the sign described by Ortolani (1948) as an outward rotation of the legs in the new-born with preluxation of the hip joints in the "position of abandonment".

Plagiocephaly. Moulding of the foetal skull by the uterus has been observed by many previous authorities, and a paediatrician in New York was said to diagnose CDH by simply observing the heads of his new-born lying in their cots. Such moulding often takes the form of plagiocephaly, which involves the flattening of one side of the anterior half of the skull. It is uncommon in normal cephalic deliveries and this is thought to be due to the fact that the head has previously been protected by the maternal pelvis

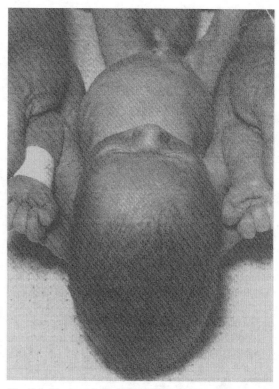

Fig. 5.5. Plagiocephaly (right-sided). Right CDH in new-born. Note hollow in right adductor region. Same new-born as in Fig. 5.10.

during the last stages of pregnancy. The moulding of the head at birth is seen in Fig. 5.5.

In the Southampton survey, it was found in 4% of normal breech deliveries when the skull had remained in contact with the fundus of the uterus for some weeks before birth. The degree of deformity was greater in 30% of new-born with reducible hip displacements, and it was still more obvious in 50% of those with irreducible hip displacements. When the CDH was unilateral the plagiocephaly was on the side of displacement, but in bilateral cases it was usually on the left. One new-born had a marked degree of plagiocephaly associated with a facial palsy on the same side, and another developed a sternomastoid tumour and later torticollis on the same side of hip displacement.

Dunn (1976) described dolichocephaly as a typical longitudinal moulding of both sides of the foetal skull caused by the fundus of the uterus in children with CDH, but this has been a rare finding in our series. Chapple and Davidson (1941) described similar signs of pressure on the mouth and jaws of new-born due to contact with the shoulder or the feet of the foetus, sometimes in association with torticollis, but they did not mention moulding of the skull.

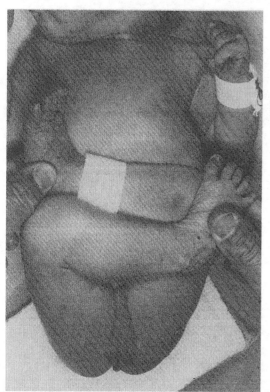

Fig. 5.4. The position of dislocation, identified in nearly every new-born with CDH. Note the excessive lateral rotation of the flexed thigh. (Wilkinson 1972, with permission)

Torticollis. The notion that congenital deformities might be caused by pressure in utero dates back at least to Hippocrates and the concept of a postural torticollis with forward displacement of the ear and occasionally an associated facial paralysis was first described by Sir Denis Browne in 1936, in his classic paper on "Congenital Deformities of Mechanical Origin". Later his ideas were developed by Hulbert (1950), who related postural torticollis to breech malposition and separated this group from the sternomastoid tumours and secondary contractures developing in infant life (see Fig. 5.6). One would have thought that there should be a close relationship between plagiocephaly, torticollis, and CDH, as found in the moulded baby syndrome described by Lloyd-Roberts and Pilcher (1965), but in our series of 400 patients many have been born with plagiocephaly, but few have had any evidence of postural torticollis, although one had a temporary facial palsy and another developed a sternomastoid tumour and contracture later on. It is surprising that the relationship is not more common, but nevertheless the presence of torticollis at birth should stimulate the examiner to scrutinise for any evidence of hip displacement, as both conditions have a common origin in breech malposition.

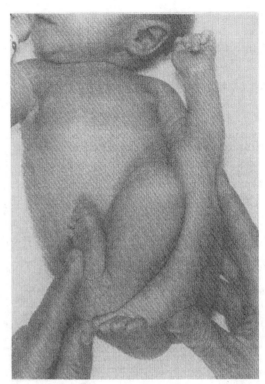

Fig. 5.7. Calcaneo-valgus moulding of right foot associated with a new-born right CDH. Such moulding should stimulate the examiner to examine the hip joint carefully.

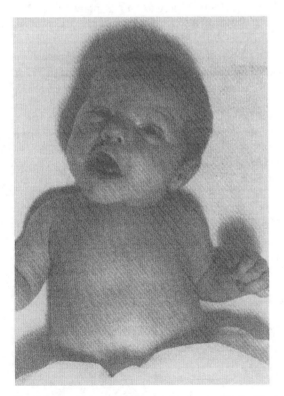

Fig. 5.6. New-born torticollis—postural, associated with right plagiocephaly, but rarely associated with CDH.

Foot Deformities. The association of a valgus moulding of the foot with CDH was first noted by Sir Denis Browne (1936). Ortolani included the same as one of his "signs of probability" in congenital luxation of the hip. Its presence at birth should always stimulate the examiner to scrutinise the hip joints more carefully. The new-born in Fig. 5.7 had an unstable hip joint. Sir Denis Browne also claimed that it was uncommon to find an equino-varus deformity of the foot, such as talipes or metatarsus varus, associated with displacement of the ipsilateral hip; but he recognised "windswept" deformities of both feet with one moulded in valgus and the other in varus, with instability of the hip joint on the side of the valgus foot, and a normal hip on the side of the varus moulding, as in Fig. 5.8. The only exception to this rule is found in cases of arthrogryphosis and neurogenic deformities of the feet associated with spina bifida. Sharrard (1968) in his studies on foot deformities associated with paralysis secondary to meningomyelocele, suggested that the intra-uterine paralysis was a predominant cause of foot deformities at birth. Reference to his tables of innervation of the lower limbs shown in Fig. 5.9 would indicate that a temporary or permanent paralysis between the levels L5 and S1 could produce a varus mould-

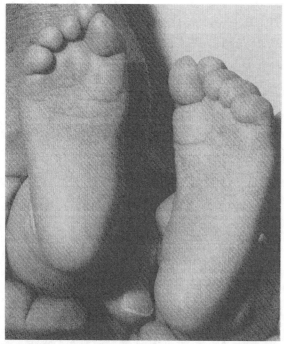

Fig. 5.8. Wind-swept feet. Right valgus and left varus moulding. The latter is rarely associated with CDH. (Same child as shown in Fig. 5.7.)

ing of the foot, due to unopposed action of the anterior and posterior tibial muscles associated with weakness of the hamstrings and the lateral rotators. Yamamuro et al. (1977) discovered in their experimental studies on the hips of female rats that with the knee joint immobilised in extension the hip failed to dislocate spontaneously when the hamstrings were divided!

When the paralysis is more peripheral, occurring between the S1 and S2 level, it will affect the long flexors of the toes and the intrinsic muscles of the feet, leaving the dorsiflexors and evertors to become dominant, associated with some innervation of the hamstrings and lateral rotators. This would result in a calcaneovalgus moulding of the foot and muscle power sufficient to rotate laterally the flexed hip joint, contributing to the mechanism of displacement. Such levels of permanent paralysis can be mimicked by temporary paralysis, as suggested by Drachman and Coulombre (1962), and explain the relationship of foot moulding to hip displacement in utero.

Signs of Hip Displacement

There are three classic groups of signs, which provide indisputable evidence of hip displacement when two or more are positive. Their presence is

LEVEL OF INNERVATION	PROGRESSIVE INNERVATION OF FOOT MUSCLES	MUSCULAR ACTION	
Lumbar 4 5	Tibialis anterior Tibialis posterior	Dorsiflexion Inversion	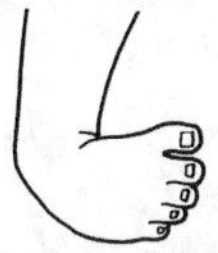 Calcaneo-varus
Sacral 1	Peroneus brevis Peroneus longus	Eversion	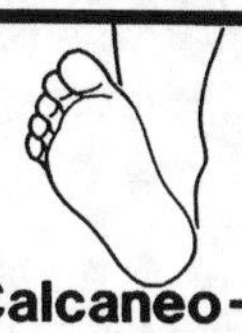 Calcaneo-valgus
2	Gastrocnemius Soleus	Plantar flexion	Equino varus
3	Flexor digitorum Foot intrinsics	Inversion	

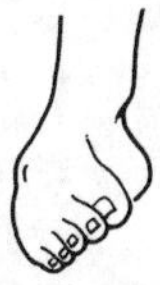

Fig. 5.9. Sharrard's table of innervation. Progressive innervation in a cranio-caudal direction produces these changes in foot posture.

dependent upon the degree of displacement and whether the hip is reducible. Leg inequality is dependent upon one leg being normal, or near normal, and may not exist in bilateral cases. Limitation of abduction may be absent in the reducible hip, but is usually present in the irreducible displacement except in patients with extreme degrees of joint laxity. Hip instability is foolproof evidence of hip displacement, but it may be very difficult to detect in those that are irreducible.

Leg Inequality. At birth displacement is less frequently unilateral than bilateral (Palmen 1961; MacKenzie 1972), but there is usually a degree of inequality in bilateral displacements, depending upon whether both hips are equally displaced, and overt inequality is always present in unilateral displacements. Above-knee shortening is always more apparent with both hips and knees flexed as in Fig. 5.10, as this posture tends to displace the unstable hip. Adduction and medial rotation of the thighs also aggravate displacement, making the inequality more pronounced. Above-knee shortening of the thigh often produces inequality of the medial skin folds, seen in Fig. 5.11, the asymmetry being due to the deeper and more proximal folds on the side of displacement. The sign is also evident when the new-born is lying prone and one observes the gluteal fold, as the latter is raised on the side of displacement (see Fig. 5.14). The signs are more apparent in new-born with total displacement of the hip, and become more distinct in all cases by the sixth week of life owing to the deposition of sub-

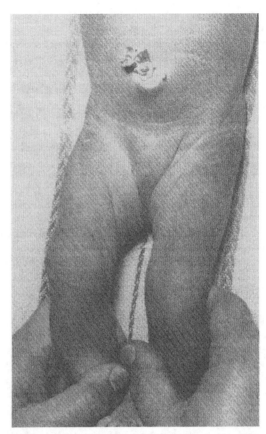

Fig. 5.11. New-born with right CDH. Note above-knee shortening and unequal skin folds in adductor region. (Wilkinson 1972, with permission)

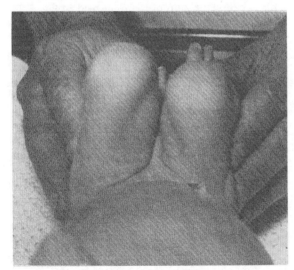

Fig. 5.10. Above-knee leg shortening, right CDH at birth. Note the shallow impression in the adductors. Same new-born as in Fig. 5.5. (Wilkinson 1972, with permission)

cutaneous fat. When the new-born lies supine, the inguinal fold on the side of displacement tends to conceal the vulva. This is partly due to the fact that the affected leg is held quietly in partial flexion, whereas the other leg moves freely (Chapple and Davidson 1941).

The Snapping Sign of Hip Instability. This is the most uncontroversial sign of pre-natal hip displacement in the new-born, but in order to demonstrate it clearly one must have the baby completely relaxed. This can be attained in the supine position by flexing her hips and knees fully, creating the position of comfort which relaxes the child sufficiently to allow the examiner to undertake his critical assessment. This fully flexed posture also rotates the acetabulum in an anticlockwise direction to bring the defect in the acetabular rim into the postero-inferior position (Weinberg and Pogrund 1980). The examiner stabilises the pelvis by holding one of the hips flexed on the abdomen, with one hand, in order to examine the opposite hip with his free hand. On this side, he

places the middle finger on the greater trochanter
laterally and the thumb on the adductor aspect of
the thigh medially. Pressure under the tip of the
greater trochanter lifts the femoral head into the
acetabulum over the posterior rim and it can be felt
to jerk into the socket. Then release of the index
finger allows the femoral head to fall downward out
of the acetabulum with a similar sensation. This test
is as described by Roser (1864) and Le Damany
(1914), and is very similar to the provocative tests
of Palmen (1948) and Barlow (1962).

When there is no obstruction to concentric reduction, the "snapping" sensation is very clear and distinct; but if there is a small incarcerated limbus, the
femoral head may be felt to roll over the posterior
rim and the sensation is more muffled and indistinct.
If the limbus is large and there is an associated contracture of the anterior capsule, the test will be negative, even in the presence of complete displacement,
as demonstrated in Fig. 5.12.

Limitation of Abduction. Ortolani (1948) described
two separate signs based on this feature of hip displacement at birth; one with the patient lying
supine and the other prone. In the supine position
with thighs flexed and hips abducted there is a
greater resistance on the involved side and sometimes a cavity forms in the adductor fold. This is the
sign of Joachimisthl, shown in Fig. 5.13. With the
patient lying in the prone position, abduction of the
legs with the hips in extension usually reveals
limited abduction on the side of displacement even
when the hip is reducible. Also the more proximal
portion of the thigh, or the upper surface, appears

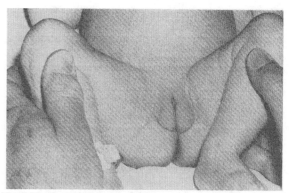
Fig. 5.13. Limited abduction left hip—supine. Left CDH.

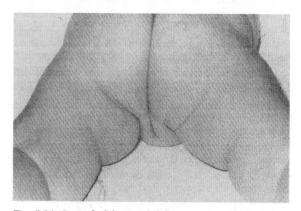
Fig. 5.14. Limited abduction left hip—prone. Left CDH. Same patient as Fig. 5.13.

to be more pronounced than on the healthy side.
This is called the sign of Delitala, seen in Fig. 5.14.
Chapple and Davidson (1941) described the sign of
limited abduction, as one of the predominant signs
of hip displacement after the initial relaxation of the
new-born infant had disappeared. They believed it
to be due to the splinting of the unstabilised femoral
head by its surrounding muscles. Palmen (1961)
also described it as an important sign in the new-
born, but found it unusual in the more common preluxations and suggested it should arouse suspicion
of complete luxation if observed in a child who was
otherwise relaxed.

Von Rosen (1962) believed that such limitation
of abduction was a post-natal development occurring after the first 2 days of life, and was due to the
development of secondary soft tissue contractures
affecting the adductor muscles. Barlow (1962) also
considered it to be a sign of delayed diagnosis. Yet
many other authorities have observed this sign at
birth, believing it to be a pre-natal development in
the presence of hip displacement.

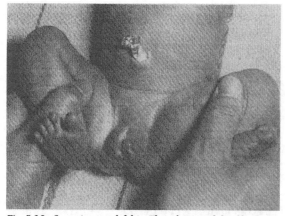
Fig. 5.12. Snapping test, left hip. The pelvis is stabilised by flexing
the opposite hip fully and grasping the pelvis between thumb and
fingers. The left thigh is then held lightly, between the thumb
and fingers as a pen, and "waggled" gently. The head of the femur
can be felt to jump in and out of the socket!

In the Southampton survey (Wilkinson 1972), 1 in 1000 live births revealed all the features of breech malposition and hip displacement, including leg inequality and limitation of abduction, without there being any evidence of the snapping sign on the day they were born. Similar experience was recorded by MacKenzie (1972), who stated that "congenital dislocation of the hip may first present as either instability or as limitation of abduction. The latter may accompany or replace instability, or rarely instability may replace stiffness." This is in keeping with Ortolani's original observation that "stiff hips at birth, when splinted with an abduction pillow, can develop instability within the first few weeks of life".

Radiological Features of CDH in the New-born

Even the most enthusiastic observers admit that orthodox radiographs of the new-born are frequently difficult to assess, as there are many causes for error in judgement. This is mainly because the proximal femoral epiphysis is not apparent at birth and one is forced to measure the relationship between the ossified parts of the proximal femoral metaphysis and the pelvis. Sometimes there is no doubt about the presence of displacement when this is excessive, as shown in the irreducible hip displacement X-rayed in Fig. 5.15. In reducible hips the diagnosis is dependent upon the femoral head being displaced outside the acetabulum and the radiological findings are negative if spontaneous reduction has taken place beforehand. In other

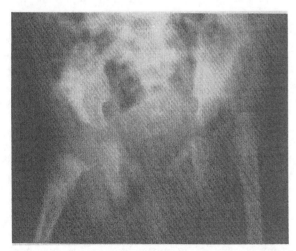

Fig. 5.15. X-ray at 2 weeks, total intra-uterine displacement of left hip. This is very obvious even in the absence of proximal femoral epiphyses.

words it is necessary to displace the femoral head in order to obtain a positive radiograph (Palmen 1961). Thus most authorities agree that clinical examination, including the snapping sign of Ortolani, is far more conclusive of hip instability than any radiological assessment and one should only depend upon the latter in those patients where the Ortolani sign is negative (MacKenzie 1972).

Acetabular Dysplasia. Putti (1933) was the first to claim to be able to diagnose the state of pre-dislocation of the hip joint radiologically at birth and stressed the necessity of submitting every new-born child to routine radiological examination. He was convinced that in those cases where radiographs revealed acetabular dysplasia, treatment at the very moment of observation, even if it be on the first day of birth, would guarantee a cure in 95% of cases. He did, however, recognise the rarer form of "embryonary hip joints" that were completely dislocated before birth, but considered them to be rare compared to the commoner pre-dislocation hip that tended to become a complete dislocation post-natally. Variations in the acetabular angles were previously reported by Hilgenreiner (1925) and later by Faber (1937) and were considered to be a radiological sign of hip displacement.

Caffey et al. in 1956 failed to find any radiological evidence of congenital dysplasia of the acetabulum to support Putti's pre-dislocation hypothesis as the common cause of post-natal dislocation. Palmen (1961) showed that rotation of the pelvis in both the sagittal plane and from side to side affected the acetabular angle, and he came to the conclusion that the measurement had no significance unless it was known that the child had been kept in a symmetrical position. He found that the measurement of straight antero-posterior radiographs of the pelvis only revealed evidence of hip displacement in 50% of new-born with positive Ortolani signs.

Andren's Radiological Test. Andren and Von Rosen (1958) described a method in which the child's legs were abducted to about 40° and extended and fully medially rotated. In this position they found that the longitudinal axis of the femur normally points to the bony edge of the acetabulum, but when the femoral head is displaced the same line often points as high as the antero-superior iliac spine, as demonstrated in Fig. 5.16. They agreed however that such measurements were only of diagnostic value in hips that were clinically unstable and had little value in patients with a negative Ortolani sign. They came to the conclusion that the radiological diagnosis of dislocation of the hip was only of secondary importance compared to the clinical findings.

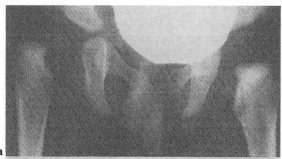

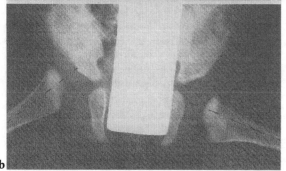

Fig. 5.16a,b. New-born right CDH, radiology. a AP film. Right hip displacement apparent, but left hip suspect. b Andren's view—note line along shaft of right femur is projected above the outer angle of acetabulum, whereas a similar line along the left femur is well within the acetabulum. Both Ortolani signs positive, right persisted.

Andren (1962) also described another radiological test to demonstrate pelvic instability. Two radiographs were taken with the legs in 90° of abduction and flexion, one with the femurs pushed towards each other and the other when they were pulled apart. The symphysis pubis was measured and also the greatest distance between the lateral outlines of the two ischial bones, plus the distances between the outlines of the ossified parts of the ends of the femurs. He came to the conclusion that there was a definite degree of pelvic instability in the new-born, but it had wide individual variations. It was more marked in females than males and was more pronounced in new-born with congenital hip displacement, being somewhat greater in bilateral than in unilateral cases.

MacKenzie (1972) agreed with Barlow (1968) that radiological examination was unnecessary and might even be misleading in the diagnosis of CDH. The various tests described by Andren and Von Rosen were tried in patients with and without instability. They were found to be positive in 63% of unstable hips but only 30% of stiff hips. More recently Bertol et al. (1982) in Edinburgh devised standard antero-posterior radiographs of the pelvis in new-born and measured the separation between the proximal end of the femur and the pelvic wall. They found this to be significantly increased in cases of unilateral and bilateral hip displacements, there being a medial gap greater than 5 mm to indicate femoral head displacement. They found the test to be helpful when the clinical diagnosis was uncertain, but even with this investigation the rate of missed dislocations was 0.6 cases per 1000, which is nearer to the figure of persistent hip displacement in the untreated population. Although they proposed the use of radiographs as an aid to diagnosis in CDH, they were forced to agree that it was controversial, yet found the method of value in those cases where clinical diagnosis was in doubt.

Neonatal Displacement Between 1 and 10 Months

During this early phase of post-natal life the diagnosis of CDH becomes more difficult both clinically and radiologically, as evidence of hip instability disappears while that of persistent displacement becomes more apparent. All the difficulties encountered in the radiological diagnosis at birth persist until the proximal femoral epiphyses appear, but this can be delayed until after the neonatal period.

Some of the affected children are picked up at birth with all the evidence of CDH, but fail to respond to treatment and either remain unstable or develop limitation of abduction. Other patients are referred from infant welfare clinics at 3–4 months, because of leg inequality or limitation of abduction affecting one or both thighs.

Clinical Signs

One must be aware of the disappearing signs of breech malposition as described in the new-born, for plagiocephaly, torticollis, scoliosis, and calcaneovalgus deformity of the feet may persist either in isolation or together as in the "moulded baby syndrome" (Lloyd-Roberts and Pilcher 1965). In addition the signs of persistent hip displacement usually become more apparent within the first few months of life.

Asymmetry of the Folds of the Thighs. Although this sign is said to be misleading in the new-born (Palmen 1961) persistent asymmetry becomes more obvious as the child grows and the gluteal and inguinal folds become more evident (Ortolani 1948), as shown in Figs. 5.17 and 5.18.

Flattening of the Buttock. This is an important sign which is more obvious in unilateral cases than in bilateral CDH. It is visible when the child is lying in the prone position and becomes more prominent

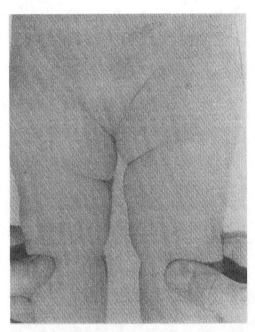

Fig. 5.17. Neonatal left CDH (4 months). There is above-knee shortening and the unequal skin creases are more prominent due to increased subcutaneous fat.

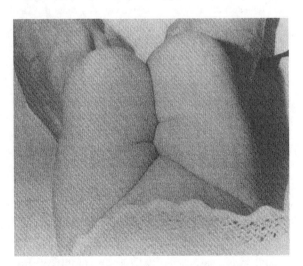

Fig. 5.18. Neonatal left CDH (4 months). The above-knee shortening is more apparent with hips flexed, and the same can be said for the unequal adductor folds. (Same child as shown in Fig. 5.17.)

as the natural gluteal fat disappears. Wasting of the buttock can sometimes be appreciated more by palpation with the flat of the palm than by observing the contour of the buttock.

Raised Greater Trochanter. This can be detected with the child lying supine with both legs extended. The examiner places his thumbs on the anterior superior iliac spines and his index fingers on the tips of the greater trochanters. Inequality of height makes the raised trochanter more obvious in unilateral cases, but displacement can also be detected in bilateral cases after long experience. The test is demonstrated in Fig. 6.3.

Limited Abduction. This has been carefully described in the new-born, but the sign becomes more prominent in persistent hip displacement, especially when inequality appears in unilateral cases. With the patient lying in the supine position and both hips flexed, abduction of one or both thighs meets greater resistance on the affected side and sometimes a cavity appears in the adductor fold, as seen in Fig. 5.19. When the patient is lying prone, abduction is also limited on the side of displacement and the outer aspect of the proximal portion of the thigh becomes more prominent than on the healthy side (Ortolani 1948).

The Scatto or "Snapping" Sign. Instability of the hip can persist in 13% of cases during the first 3 months of life (MacKenzie 1972), and Ortolani (1948) suggested that such a persistence gave a poor prognosis. The sign is more difficult to demonstrate in this age group, as the children resist examination and they also appear to experience discomfort during the procedure, which makes further examnation either difficult or impossible. In some patients when the sign

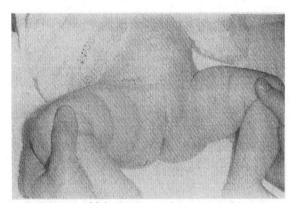

Fig. 5.19. Neonatal left CDH (4 months). Limited abduction of left hip. Note that the left thigh is higher than the right in relation to the body. (Same child as shown in Fig. 5.17.)

is negative on routine clinical examination, a general anaesthetic restores the instability, indicating that it has been masked by muscle guarding rather than contracture. When a contracture is present, an adductor tenotomy sometimes restores the snapping sign (Wilkinson 1975).

Apparent Hip Displacement. In their paper on the pitfalls in the management of CDH, Lloyd-Roberts and Swann (1966) described an apparent clinical form of hip displacement in patients associated with concentric reduction of the hip joint. In these children the apparent above-knee shortening and limitation of abduction is due to a pelvic obliquity or lateral rotation of the affected side of the pelvis. They quoted Weissman et al. (1961), who described the same features in isolation, but added to this the "moulded baby syndrome", where the pelvic rotation was associated with plagiocephaly, torticollis, and scoliosis. The signs are identical to those of unilateral hip displacement without any clinical evidence of instability. If such children are untreated, spontaneous recovery takes place. The authors believed that no great harm is done if these patients are splinted, "unless they are unwittingly considered to exemplify successful early conservative treatment".

Radiological Signs of Neonatal Hip Displacement

As in new-born, the radiological appearances of neonatal hip displacement are confusing before the appearance of the proximal femoral epiphysis. This is because the femoral head and much of the acetabulum consists of cartilage and it is difficult to assess their relationship by orthodox radiology. Patients in whom X-rays reveal unilateral acetabular dysplasia and evidence of hip instability may recover spontaneously without treatment (see Fig. 5.20).

The age at which the proximal femoral epiphysis appears varies widely between the two sexes and in different individuals. It tends to occur earlier in girls than in boys: it can be seen in 50% of normal hips before 4 months and in 100% of female hips at 8 months, whereas in boys it can be seen in 50% at 6 months and 100% at 10 months (Yamamuro and Chen 1980). Unfortunately, the appearance is delayed in the presence of hip displacement in both sexes and may not appear in such cases until they are more than a year old. Thus a delay in the appearance of both femoral epiphyses up to the age of 12 months in either sex is of little consequence, but a

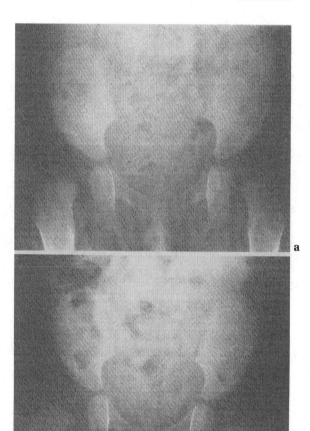

Fig. 5.20a,b. Apparent radiological displacement in neonate. **a** X-ray at 4 months. Left hip displaced due to break in Shenton's line and acetabular dysplasia. **b** X-ray of the same patient 6 months later, i.e. at 10 months, without any splinting. The epiphyses have appeared in both hips, being concentrically placed and equal. Follow-up was normal.

unilateral retardation of ossification in the proximal femoral epiphysis might well suggest some pathological condition of the hip joint regardless of its aetiology.

In apparent hip displacement, the radiological appearance may also be deceptive after the proximal femoral epiphysis is visualised, as there may be apparent superolateral displacement associated with acetabular dysplasia and also a break in Shenton's line. The tell-tale radiological evidence is a narrowing of the affected side of the pelvis involving the iliac crest, associated with an inequality of the obturator foramina. If both proximal femoral epiphyses are almost equal in size, it is unlikely that there is any displacement (see Fig. 5.21).

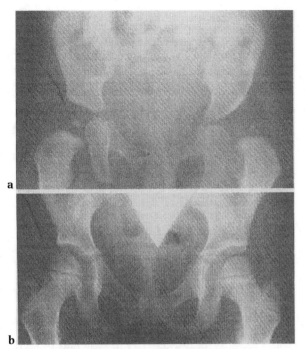

Fig. 5.21a,b. Apparent radiological displacement in neonate. **a** X-ray at 10 months. Left epiphysis not delayed in appearance and only slightly smaller than right. Shenton's line broken due to superolateral displacement? Acetabular dysplasia? but iliac crest narrower than normal side. **b** X-ray of same patient at $5\frac{1}{2}$ years. Spontaneous recovery of left hip.

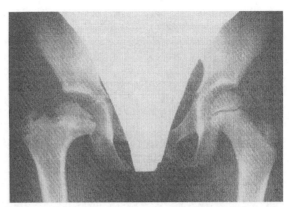

Fig. 5.22. Iatrogenic coxa plana due to splinting. At 4 months the right hip appeared displaced clinically and radiologically, but no history of instability. Treated at 4 months by examination under general anaesthesia, adductor tenotomy, and abduction splinting for 3 months. At present 2 cm above-knee shortening associated with proximal femoral epiphyseal arrest.

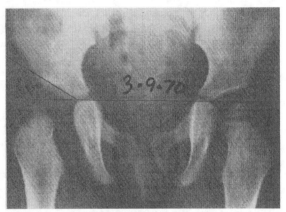

Fig. 5.23. Radiological signs, right CDH, neonate. This is the same child as in Fig. 5.16 at 10 months. The right femoral epiphysis is hypoplastic and is displaced superolaterally with a break in Shenton's line. The acetabular angle is over 30° (see charts in Chap. 6).

It is therefore difficult in new-born and neonatal patients that have above-knee shortening of the limb with limited abduction and a negative Ortolani sign, to separate clinically and radiologically those with concentrically placed femoral heads associated with pelvic obliquity and those with hip displacement. In a personal series of 78 such cases diagnosed within the first 10 months of life and not treated, 18 (23%) eventually turned out to have persistent displacement of their hips, whereas the remainder recovered spontaneously, revealing no stigmata of hip dysplasia, either clinically or radiologically, in their follow-up over a 3-year period. Previously this group were splinted in abduction and it was found that 6% of the total treated developed iatrogenic deformation of the femoral head, as shown in Fig. 5.22.

Once the epiphysis has appeared, hypoplasia of the ossific centre, compared to the opposite side, and superolateral displacement are usually pathognomonic of hip disease. When these radiological signs are associated with a unilateral acetabular dysplasia and an acetabular angle of more than 30°, the evidence indicates a congenital displacement, as seen in Fig. 5.23.

The failure of routine radiology and arthrography (Ortolani 1948) to provide a foolproof measure of ensuring indisputable evidence of hip displacement in the first 6–10 months of life has led to the exploration of many other fields of investigation, including auscultation, computed tomography, and ultrasound examinations. They are all proving to be expensive in time, effort, and equipment and their success must depend upon the degree of displacement of the femoral head at the time of examination, rather than the degree of soft tissue or bony deformation. To date, no efficient method has been discovered and it may be profitable at this stage to recall the words of George Perkins (1928), "that the diagnosis can be made and ought to be made with certainty by *inspection* alone".

Management of Normal New-born

Our attitude to this everyday problem has changed dramatically over the past 20 years in Great Britain, as in other parts of the world. Previously it was thought that the safest posture to nurse a new-born baby was on one side, in order to prevent the inhalation of vomit or regurgitation of food. It was also customary to swaddle the new-born, especially in the winter months, to prevent them from suffering from acute respiratory infections.

In the 1950s, orthopaedic and paediatric authorities began to take note of numerous reports which appeared to suggest that the nursing habits of various races throughout the world might be responsible for the production or aggravation of postural deformities. In Great Britain it was thought that the increased prevalence of persistent displacement of the hip in winter-born infants might be due to this excess swaddling in the colder season of the year (Record and Edwards 1958; Carter and Wilkinson 1964). House insulation and modern domestic heating methods have made it unnecessary to swaddle and restrict our new-born with heavy blankets during the winter months.

The growth and development of the human skeletal system is a continuous process throughout the perinatal period and the birth of a child is but an episode in the series of changes that occur. Dunn (1971) drew attention to the extremely rapid rate of growth in the foetal period and assessed it to be approximately 50 times faster than in childhood, but the rate diminishes slowly during the first 2 years of life, and half the mature length of the long bones is attained by the time the child is 6 years old. In Chap. 2 reference is made to Appleton's work which showed that persistently applied and gentle forces were sufficient to produce deformation during the rapid period of growth, and it would not be surprising if the results were similar whether they were applied either pre-natally or post-natally. Thus the nursing of the new-born must have a very important influence on the general development of the musculoskeletal system.

In most British paediatric centres we have now adopted the North American custom of nursing all babies prone from birth. It is important that they should be nursed on a thin mattress supported by a wooden base and without a pillow. Paediatricians have come to accept that this is the safest way to nurse a baby with respect to cot-deaths and it is also helpful in preventing oesophageal regurgitation. Bobath (1966) described how the new-born, full-term baby showed at rest a symmetrical attitude of flexion in all postures. Head raising in the prone position initiates a process of general extension of the trunk and limbs against gravity and this spreads in a cephalocaudal direction to reach the hips and knees around about the sixth month. This is a gradual development and spread of the normal automatic reactions for the maintenance of posture, and is a good reason for nursing new-born in this prone position.

James (1970) believed that plagiocephaly was due partly to a post-natal development and quoted a personal communication from Hay suggesting that it probably arose from lying the baby in an oblique or lateral position, the still plastic skull flowing into the shape as a result of gravity. This led him to the conclusion that gravity might similarly affect the chest and could be a cause of infantile resolving scoliosis developing in the first year of life. It has already been noted in Chap. 4, that there is a relationship between plagiocephaly and hip displacement developing pre-natally and both tend to occur on the same side. Thus these pre-natal postural deformities, due to intra-uterine position, might also be affected by a post-natal mechanism which could account for a persistence of hip displacement. MacKenzie (1972) pointed out that at birth there is a larger percentage of bilateral CDH than unilateral and whereas spontaneous recovery occurred more frequently on the right side, persistent displacement occurred on the left. This might be due to some post-natal factor, or might even be caused by the cerebral dominance of the child.

These observations sustain the belief that all new-born should be nursed prone, both night and day, from the day of birth and that the legs should be held abducted with a thick nappy or disposable diaper in order to encourage the child to flex the hips in the abducted posture. Ortolani (1948) felt that any means to limit or impede the adduction of legs would be prophylactic, and he recommended that a sturdy diaper applied in the American or English fashion might well be sufficient to stop the progression of a dysplastic hip joint. His sentiments were echoed by Palmen (1961), who noted that the instability of the hips was more common in those regions where it was customary for mothers to have their infants lying with legs straight and bound together.

Management of New-born with CDH

Adolf Lorenz (1895) was the first to advocate the principle of splinting children with CDH. His experiences with surgical reduction led him to enunciate the modern principles of conservative treatment, including the retention of the femoral head in the physiological position where it is able to exert a beneficial influence on the development of the acetabulum (Palmen 1961). Thus when Putti (1933) introduced the early diagnosis of CDH, he proposed the use of a Frejka pillow, or an adjustable divaricating splint, to abduct the legs of his patients.

Aims of Splinting

The aims of splinting include:

1) A retention of concentric reduction of the femoral head in the acetabulum during the first 6–12 weeks of life, when the maternal hormonal laxity is responsible for a temporary instability of the joint. Once the hormones have been metabolised and excreted, stability is attained and residual subluxation is unlikely to develop.

2) The stimulation of bone growth and the remodelling of the bony components of the acetabulum and femoral head, to produce congruity of the articular surfaces and resulting stability.

3) Some authorities still believe that abduction splinting can overcome soft tissue contractures and any impediment to concentric reduction caused by the interposition of capsule or limbus, without damaging the bony components as previously taught by Severin (1951).

Selection of New-born for Treatment

This has varied according to different proponents. Almost everyone would agree that it is necessary to splint the unstable hip joint in abduction, for a period long enough to ensure its stability before the child is allowed to extend and medially rotate the hips. When there is limited abduction of the hip, there are varying opinions as to whether it is wise to apply abduction splints. Palmen (1961) and Von Rosen (1968) believed that the presence of an adductor contracture was a post-natal development and indicated that the opportunity for splinting successfully had been missed, whereas MacKenzie (1972) felt that an adductor contracture was a manifestation of hip displacement and indicated the application of splints. If limitation of abduction is evidence of persistent eccentric reduction, due to the imposition of soft tissue between the femoral head and acetabular components, then enforced abduction splinting might well cause avascular necrosis due to compression of the soft femoral head. This persuaded Salter et al. (1969) to abandon the full abduction posture, at the risk of losing some element of stability, and to accept the "human" position with the hips flexed more than 90° but only slightly abducted. Putti (1933) originally advocated the application of splints for radiological dysplasia of the hip joint and there are still some who adhere to this principle in cases where the clinical diagnosis is in doubt.

Time for Splinting

This has also varied with different authorities and there is no general agreement. Putti (1933) advocated the application of splints as soon as the diagnosis had been confirmed radiologically. Ortolani (1948) proposed the early application of splints in the new-born when instability was detected, but he believed that pillows of different sizes and shapes were sufficient to stop the progression of dysplasia in the hip joint during the first months of life. Thus he did not advise the application of rigid splints during the first 3 months, but if instability persisted he used the abduction splint advocated by Putti or a plaster cast when necessary. Palmen (1961) advised splinting within the first 2 days of life, but stressed the point that the femoral head should be reduced before the application of the abduction harness. Von Rosen and more recently Fredensborg (1977) believed that the splinting should begin at birth and that a delay of more than two days might be sufficient to cause a bad result. Barlow (1962) recognised the fact that the majority of unstable hips underwent spontaneous recovery without treatment, but he eventually came to the conclusion that all should be splinted within the first week of life. MacKenzie (1972) recognised the unpopularity of early splinting with the mothers and also the fact that 50% of his cases underwent spontaneous recovery. Therefore he advocated a delay of splinting until the child was 3 weeks old. If instability persisted at that time, he applied the semi-rigid Aberdeen splint and found no evidence to prove that such a 3-week delay eventually affected the ultimate response to treatment.

If there is disagreement concerning the most effectual time to apply splints, there is generally complete agreement that they should be continued for 6–12 weeks, during which time the majority of unstable hips become stable. It is also generally accepted that if the instability persists beyond the twelfth week there is a risk to continuing with the splinting, because of the development of epiphysitis, and many of these patients eventually come to surgery (Palmen 1961).

Type of Abduction Splint

There are three popular forms today, including rigid, semi-rigid and harnesses.

Rigid splints include plaster spicas, but most modern forms are made of malleable aluminium strips such as the Von Rosen and Barlow splints. The metal is usually covered by a sponge foam or polyethylene to prevent any irritation or pressure on the baby's skin. Theoretically the problem concerning splints of this type is that they enforce rigid fixation of the hip joint, but they are the most successful in retaining stability and reduction. They appear to have the highest incidence of fragmentation (Wilkinson 1972) and another practical contra-indication is the fact that children in such splints cannot be nursed in the prone position, because of the risk of cot deaths. One is therefore forced to nurse such babies in the supine position and this creates problems itself.

Semi-rigid splints are usually made of more pliable polythene in a tubular form. MacKenzie (1972) popularised this form of splinting and it has the attraction of having no attachments above the waist. This means that the children can be nursed prone, but there is a tendency for the hips to extend beyond a right angle, allowing the femoral heads to subluxate, and therefore the efficiency of semi-rigid splints is diminished.

Pavlik (1957) introduced his harness, which has proved to be the most popular concept for abduction splinting used today. It consists of a wide chest strap with attached cross-shoulder straps, which prevent the former slipping down the trunk of the new-born. Two stirrups are attached by lateral straps both anteriorly and posteriorly, and by adjustment the stirrups hold the hips and knees flexed above a right angle. The harness allows a free range of abduction and adduction and some degree of rotation. It really prevents extension of the hips and knees and to a lesser extent adduction of the hips, these being the movements that jeopardise the stability of the hip joint. Its advocates feel that the active motion allowed in the displaced hip is guided by the harness to achieve greater stimulation, bringing about soft tissue and bony recovery. It is not dissimilar to the lively abduction splint advocated by Sir Denis Browne, but this can only be used in older children above the age of 6 months.

Southampton Management

In 1965 the author was entrusted with the care of a captive population of 375 000 with an average birth rate of 6000. An early attempt was made to fulfil the promises made by Von Rosen and Barlow, aimed at eliminating persistent CDH in the population. Nevertheless cases of persistent displacement continued to be discovered in the infant age group and the prevalence remained at 0.7 per 1000 normal births (McKeown and Record 1951). Half of these infant cases had been carefully examined by their doctors at birth and passed as normal. Apart from the failure to detect these cases, there was also the disturbing fact that there were some that were recognised at birth, but failed to respond to immediate splinting, and in others the treatment had produced iatrogenic deformity affecting the growth of the proximal end of the femur and acetabulum.

In 1968 it was decided to undertake a complete and comprehensive study of the problem over a 12-month period, in the hope of perfecting an early method of diagnosis in order to eliminate the missed cases and also select those that would prove resistant to early splinting. The results were reviewed and published (Wilkinson 1972). Out of 6272 live births there were 23 new-born with positive Ortolani signs, nine having bilateral instability. Barlow splints were applied at birth and the stability of the hips was checked on the tenth day (see Fig. 5.24). When the hips remained unstable the

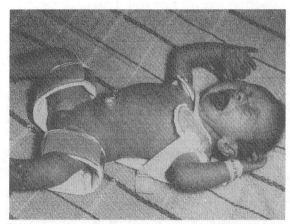

Fig. 5.24. Barlow splint made of malleable aluminium strips covered by polyethylene.

splints were retained for 8–12 weeks and this was followed up by a long-term observation. Generally the results were excellent and only three hips revealed minor degrees of dysplasia, none of which required subsequent surgical treatment, as seen in Fig. 5.25.

There were also six new-born revealing all the clinical signs of hip displacement, but with negative Ortolani signs. They were diagnosed at birth, and another six with very similar features were picked up within the first 4 months after birth, and two were discovered later. Except for the last two cases, the 12 were all treated in abduction splints, but 50% failed to respond to treatment and came to surgery, plus the two who presented later. In the patients who came to surgery it was discovered that persistent eccentric reduction of the femoral head was due to an incarceration of the limbus formed by a posterior fold of capsule, as demonstrated in Fig. 5.26. Unfortunately they all retained the stigmata of their early neonatal splinting with late deformation of the femoral epiphysis and some residual coxa plana, seen in Fig. 5.27. Three developed persistent femoral shortening due to a disturbance in the proximal femoral growth, and of

these, two came to femoral lengthening when they were 10 years old as their residual leg shortening was more than 5 cm. These iatrogenic deformities caused the rejection of rigid splinting in new-born, and it was agreed that all should be nursed in a prone posture both night and day and those with hip instability should be nursed with a large thick double nappy or disposable diaper in order to prevent adduction and extension of the child's leg during the first 3 months of life. This management was continued from 1972 to 1980.

In a retrospective review of all patients with CDH born in Southampton between 1965 and 1978, my colleagues George Bennet and John Catford assessed the outcome of management. Previous to 1972 there were 52 new-born with persistent hip instability that were treated on rigid splints, and after 1972 there were another 50 new-born with persistent hip instability that were treated with double nappies combined with prone lying. In those treated on rigid splints 92% stabilised, but the remainder remained unstable and 8% of those that stabilised developed moderate or severe epiphysitis of the affected joint, making an overall failure rate of 16%. Of those treated subsequently by prone lying

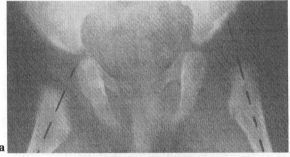

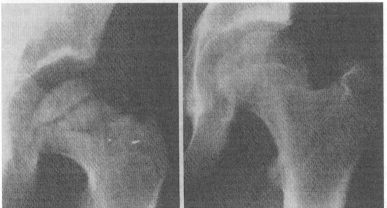

Fig. 5.25a–c. Iatrogenic deformity resulting from rigid splinting at birth. **a** New born girl with left positive Ortolani test. Treated from birth, Barlow splint for 12 weeks. X-ray at 6 weeks—hip remained unstable, but at 12 weeks Ortolani sign negative. **b** X-ray at 4 years shows metaphyseal changes. **c** X-ray at 12 years—mild coxa valga. (Wilkinson 1975, with permission)

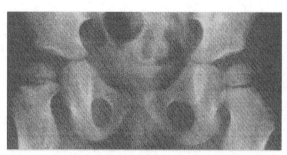

Fig. 5.26. Persistent eccentric reduction due to incarcerated limbus. First-born boy with bilateral Ortolani test positive at birth. Treated in semi-rigid abduction splint for 6 weeks; at the end of this time both hips were stable. X-ray at 18 months revealed metaphyseal changes in right hip. (Wilkinson 1975, with permission)

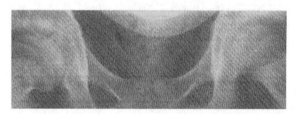

Fig. 5.27. Radiological stigmata of epiphyseal compression at birth. Same patient as in Fig. 5.26 at 12 years. There is a loss of epiphyseal height in the right hip, with a slight degree of coxa plana.

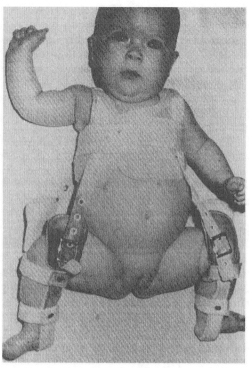

Fig. 5.28. Pavlik harness. It is essential for the hips to be flexed above 90°.

and double nappies, 50% stabilised and required no further treatment, but the others persisted and came to surgery. Yet none of this series developed avascular necrosis. Before making a critical comparison of these two series, it must be pointed out that they were consecutive and therefore could not be considered identical, as the experience of the author during the period made the second series of patients far more selective and possibly more resistant to their early management. If however it is accepted that 50% of persistent hip displacements in the general population are missed at birth, then early treatment can only involve the remaining 50%.

As half of those splinted would undergo spontaneous recovery with simple nursing techniques, only 50% will persist if not splinted. If 16% of this remnant either fail to stabilise or develop epiphysitis as a result of splinting, it means that only 34% will benefit from early splinting. Thus early diagnosis and management can only prevent the minority of persistent CDH developing in the general population. This might explain why there is little to convince that all the efforts of diagnosis at birth and early treatment have made much impression, if any,

upon the prevalence of this increasing problem of persistent CDH in our community.

Although it was pleasing to see that the rejection of rigid splints at birth meant that no new-born was subsequently damaged by treatment, the higher prevalence of persistent instability was a source of concern, and so in 1980 it was decided to undertake a new programme. Since then all new-born have been examined, and those with instability, as well as limitation of abduction and leg inequality, have been indexed and subjected to follow-up. Each patient has been nursed in the prone position both night and day, and when instability has been detected clinically, the legs are held abducted and flexed with double nappies. If hip instability persists at 3 weeks, the hips are splinted in abduction and flexion above a right angle, by the application of a Pavlik harness (see Fig. 5.28). This is maintained until stability is established, but the splints are not retained beyond 12 weeks. The results of this prospective study are not yet available, but to date there has been little difference between the outcome of children treated previously by prone lying and double nappies, and those that have been splinted subsequently. Only two children treated in a Pavlik harness have developed any evidence of epiphysitis and this has been mild. Those neonates that have persistent hip instability after 12 weeks of splinting, have been allowed to kick free and encouraged to lie prone both night and day. All have come to surgical management at the age of 10 months and the majority have been found to have an incarcerated limbus in the eccentrically reduced or unstable hip joints. It is known that a similar management was surveyed by Suzuki (1979), and he found an 83% success rate, the remainder either failing to stabilise or developing deformity of the femoral head secondary to epiphysitis. It is hoped to prevent such complications in the present series by accepting three main contra-indications to splinting at 3 weeks of age:

1) Moderate or severe limitation of abduction of the affected hip joint

2) Instability of reduction and inability to maintain the femoral head in the acetabulum

3) A "muffled" or indistinct Ortolani test

For these are the clinical signs of eccentric reduction and indicate that a limbus is present. Such cases are nursed prone with a double nappy and observed for the next 10 months, it being accepted that many will come to surgery.

Other Series

Palmen (1961), Von Rosen (1962), and Barlow (1962) discovered instability in the hips of newborn in 2.2, 1.7, and 1.55 per 1000 live births respectively. They all advised the application of rigid splints within 2–3 days of birth and claimed an 80%–90% excellent response to this treatment over a period not greater than 12 weeks. Yet they accepted the fact that spontaneous recovery might have taken place in 50% or more of these cases without treatment, and in the 10%–20% of those that failed to develop normal hip joints there was persistent subluxation, acetabular dysplasia, or femoral head deformation. Retrospectively Palmen claimed to have lowered the prevalence of persistent infantile dislocation in his newborn population from 85% before 1955, to 23% after 1960 as a result of his management. But it must be pointed out that this prevalence of persistent infantile CDH is only half that discovered in Southampton when newborn were treated with double nappies and prone lying, and there was no morbidity in the Southampton series.

When reviewing the success of management in previously published series, it is necessary to ask one very important question: is the author claiming the outcome of treatment of hip instability, or is he assessing the treatment of all abnormal hips at birth, i.e. those with instability and those with stiffness with or without instability? Palmen, Von Rosen, and Barlow believed that limitation of abduction and a negative Ortolani test only resulted from postnatal changes and were manifestations of late presentation; therefore they excluded these cases from their series and only assessed the results of treatment in those patients with frank instability of their joints. This means that they were selecting those patients who were likely to recover spontaneously or respond to simple treatment. Perhaps MacKenzie (1972) published the most extensive survey of new-born in a captive population in Great Britain, in which he included abnormal hips that were unstable and also those with limited abduction with or without instability. He claimed that 1 in 50 of normal births were born with abnormal hips, two thirds being unstable and one third having only stiffness. Half the total recovered spontaneously within the first 3 weeks of life and he delayed his splinting until after this time. His failure rate was 5% and the majority of those required surgical treatment later. The prevalence of these failed cases was 0.5 per 1000 of the population, which approaches the prevalence reported by Record and Edwards. A similar experience stimulated Noble et al. (1978) to write:

Despite earlier optimism about the ease and accuracy of diagnosing congenital dislocation of the hips in newborn babies, it has since become clear that some are still being missed during neonatal screening examinations. There is also increasing recognition that the routine treatment of unstable hips in the newborn, many cases of which would correct spontaneously, may itself cause ischaemic damage to the femoral head if incorrectly applied.

Perhaps Ortolani (1978) should have the last word, for in a letter to *The Lancet* in correspondence he wrote:

I agree with you that screening for hip dislocation in the neonatal department alone "is inadequate protection against future disability". However this "inadequate protection" should not be due to failure of diagnosis but only to treatment which is still not always successful even when started at an early age by experienced staff.

In my experience a consistently negative click (jerk) test since birth accompanied by normal abduction of the thighs reflects a normal hip or a simple dysplasia which will recover spontaneously. On the other hand, a negative clinical test with very limited abduction makes a congenital pelvic deformity or severe dislocation very likely, and suggests the need for an X-ray. . . .

Dislocation of the hip will long remain a challenge to the patience and skill of the orthopaedic team.

Thus a review of some of the leading series of patients treated by the advocates of early diagnosis and neonatal splinting suggests that all their efforts are not reducing significantly the percentage of the population that are requiring in-patient treatment for persistent displacement of the hips in infantile life.

Failure of Treatment

It was shown in Chap. 4 that the prevalence of persistent CDH in the infant population after the first 10 months has not diminished as a result of screening new-born babies and treating them at birth or within the first few weeks of life, and in any community the abolition of persistent cases must be the final judgement of the effectiveness of neonatal screening and treatment. Von Rosen (1968) in Malmö claimed to have reduced the incidence of infant CDH to 0.07 per 1000 live births, and Mitchell (1972) in Edinburgh at one time claimed a similar prevalence of 0.13, but this has subsequently been increased to 0.6 cases per 1000 live births (Bertol et al. 1982). Mackenzie (1972) in Aberdeen had a prevalence of 0.91, whereas in Southampton the figure was 1.27. These last three figures surround that of 0.65 per 1000 live births of infantile dislocation published by Record and Edwards (1958) in Birmingham, long before neonatal screening was introduced into this country. Place et al. (1978) in Leeds stated that "despite the examination of neonates for congenital dislocation of the hip, this condition is being diagnosed after the new-born period at a rate not very different from that reported before the introduction of screening". They suggested that the figures implied (1) some infants are not tested at birth, (2) the tester is unable to detect all cases, and (3) the defect can arise after the new-born period. They dismissed the third alternative, as they could find no evidence of CDH occurring de novo after the new-born period, as previously reported by Barlow (1962). They concluded there was no escape from the fact that routine testing had a substantial false negative rate. It must also be remembered that Palmen recorded

that 10% of preluxations, which might be expected to develop into dislocations later on in life, escape diagnosis at birth.

Added to this prevalence of missed cases are the number of new-born with positive signs of hip instability or displacement that fail to respond to abduction splinting, which amounts to at least another 10%–20% (Palmen 1961; Von Rosen 1968). Previously Ortolani (1948) recognised the persistence of the snapping sign during the period of treatment and suggested that this was of poor prognosis. In our experience the persistence of instability in splinted patients is not a rare phenomenon, as demonstrated in Fig. 5.29. For instance a girl born in February 1969, by breech delivery, to a primigravid mother was found to have marked instability of both hips, the Ortolani test being positive on each side. There were no signs of adductor contractures on either side and a full range of passive abduction in both hips was easily attained. On reduction the left hip felt stable, but the right was very unstable. When the hip was held in flexion and abduction the femoral head could be felt to slip in and out of the socket with minimal movement. A Barlow abduction rigid splint was applied without force and retained for 6 weeks. By the end of this time the left hip had stabilised, but the right one remained unstable. Splinting was continued for a further 6 weeks, but the right hip failed to stabilise, as shown in Fig. 5.30. It was then accepted that persistent instability was due to eccentric reduction of the femoral head and it was decided that it would be unwise to continue the splinting under these circumstances. When the child was 6 months old, arthrography was performed (Fig. 5.30) and this demonstrated eccentric reduction of the right femoral head due to an infolded limbus. Eventually

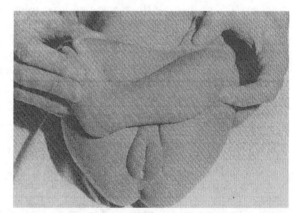

Fig. 5.29. Birth posture associated with bilateral hip instability. First-born, breech delivery. The same patient as in Figs. 5.16 and 5.23.

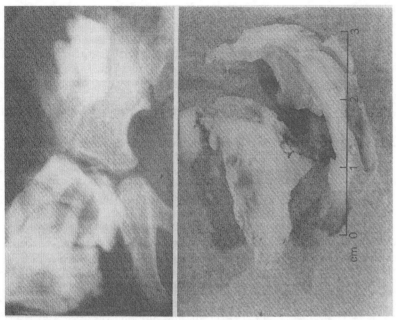

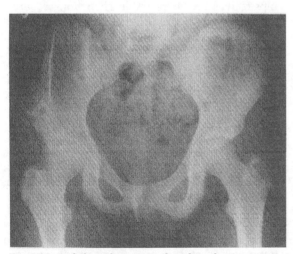

a   b

Fig. 5.30a,b. Eccentric reduction due to incarcerated limbus. **a** Arthrogram, at 12 months, in patient shown in Fig. 5.29. **b** Limbus, two layers, removed through posterior arthrotomy. (Wilkinson 1975, with permission)

Fig. 5.31. Radiological stigmata of epiphyseal compression at birth. The same patient as in Fig. 5.30, having had a pelvic osteotomy at 3 years. X-ray at 14 years revealed a slight degree of residual coxa plana in right hip. (Wilkinson 1975, with permission)

she came to surgery and the limbus was removed through a posterior arthrotomy, allowing concentric reduction of the hip to take place. Although her abduction splinting was continued for 6 months post-operatively, eventually it was found necessary to perform a pelvic osteotomy in order to correct the residual dysplasia. A recent X-ray at the age of 14 revealed the results of her early treatment. It can be seen that she retained the stigmata of epiphyseal compression in her right hip. We now have numerous examples of similar cases that have been diagnosed at birth and treated with rigid or semi-rigid splints, as well as Pavlik harnesses, but have failed to stabilise owing to the fact that reduction of the hip had been eccentric from the very beginning because of the incarceration of a limbus. Such a case is shown in Fig. 5.32 and was reported previously by Wilkinson (1975).

Neonatal CDH Response to Treatment

There is no subject in orthopaedic surgery that is likely to arouse greater emotion and diversity of opinion than the management of a child with a CDH that has first been diagnosed at 3 months of age. The strong impulse to treat as soon as the diagnosis is made, is fuelled with the challenge of delayed treatment and all its complications, and the knowledge that the morbidity of early treatment may not be revealed until many years later. Yet there are two insurmountable difficulties. The first is the confirmation of diagnosis before the appearance of the proximal femoral epiphysis; the second is the

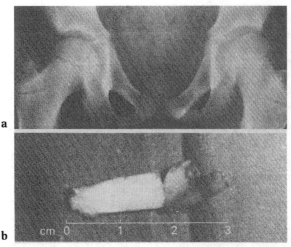

a

b

Fig. 5.32a,b. Failure of splinting at birth. **a** X-ray of 6-year-old, first-born girl. Left hip unstable at birth and splinted in a Pavlik harness for 8 weeks. Subsequent stiffness of left hip, later to become painful. Radiological evidence of left acetabular dysplasia and subluxation. **b** Incarcerated limbus excised by arthrotomy, at the time of pelvic osteotomy, which was followed by a loss of pain and full recovery.

inherent susceptibility of the proximal femoral epiphysis to permanent mechanical damage in the first 6 months of life (Kalamchi and MacEwen 1980). Thus the younger surgeon is fired with the ideal of early management, but the wiser and older colleague who has reaped the reward of early enthusiasm is inclined to wait. In the words of an old mentor, to a young mother with a 3-month-old child having a CDH, "bring her back when she is a year old and I will guarantee to cure her".

In Southampton, 20 years of experience has proved that there is no safe method of treatment in the first 10 months of life, unless one is certain that an eccentric position is not enforced upon the hip joint during reduction and subsequent splinting. The risk of severe forms of avascular necrosis cannot be eliminated. We have tried tenotomy and traction and various forms of splintage without consistent success. There has not been any encouragement to rule out eccentric reduction by arthrography at this age, with the principle of initiating our successful infantile management earlier in the neonatal period, because the results of patients first presenting between 10 and 18 months remain so good, as reported in Chap. 6.

Tonnis (1982) found in the conservative management of CDH, in the first 2 years of life, that the occurrence of necrosis of the femoral head was not dependent on the age of the patient. In cases where open reduction was attempted, without any previous closed reduction of the femoral head, not only

was there no age dependence established but the percentage of necrosis did not increase with the severity of the dislocation. He quoted Moraki and his associates in Athens (1973), who were of the opinion that after the third month of life open reduction is indicated for virtually every case of genuine dislocation of the hip. Tonnis himself believed that open reduction prior to the eighteenth month of life was indicated when conservative reduction failed, or when the reduction was incomplete and the femoral head was not concentrically seated within the acetabulum due to interposed soft tissues. In these instances, the reduction is so unstable that retention is ensured only in extreme and forced positions of the thighs. Moraki (1973) performed 117 open reductions between the third and twelfth months of age and observed an incidence of necrosis no higher than 3%.

Chiari in 1953 treated 198 cases at ages from 3 weeks to 3 months and found that contractures had developed in 49 of the patients, forcing reduction under general anaesthesia. Of these, 21 (43%) developed a marked change in the femoral head. Even in the remaining 149 cases, in whom reduction was obtained without anaesthesia and whose hips could be easily placed in abduction because of the absence of adductor contractures, femoral changes occurred in eight, or 5% of the series. Suzuki (1979) had a similar experience treating neonates between the ages of 4 and 30 weeks with Pavlik harnesses, the results being unsatisfactory in 14.5%, of which 8.2% had deformity of the femoral heads.

In Southampton, a second-born boy with a normal birth history was found to have a marked degree of plagiocephaly affecting the left side of his head and this was associated with limitation of abduction of his left hip. There was no apparent shortening and the skin creases were equal. He was born on 18th December 1968 and it was decided not to splint him at birth, but to nurse him in the prone position with a double nappy. His hip did not improve, but at 3 months an X-ray appeared normal. At 5 months, the adductor contracture persisted and it was decided to examine his hip under anaesthesia. The hip was found to be stable even following an adductor tenotomy, which allowed full abduction of the hip joint. In order to prevent the contracture recurring he was placed in an abduction splint (Denis Browne) with his hips held in 100° of flexion and 60° of abduction, and the splint was maintained for 4 weeks. He was then allowed to kick free and kept under observation. In June 1970, when he was 18 months old, the proximal epiphysis appeared for the first time in the left hip joint and it appeared to be eccentrically placed. An arthrogram was performed, but there was no convincing evidence of eccentric reduction and so it was decided to continue to observe him for another year. In July 1971 when he was 2½ years old an X-ray showed early epiphyseal compression, as seen in Fig. 5.33. An arthrotomy was performed and an incarcerated limbus was found and excised. Ten years later, in 1981, he had a severe limp due to 5 cm of above-knee shortening of his left leg associated with instability and a positive Trendelenburg test. His X-rays revealed severe deformity of the femoral head and residual subluxation, shown in Fig. 5.34. It was

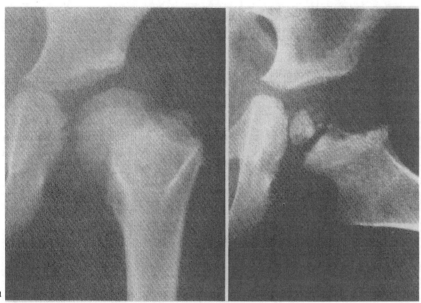

Fig. 5.33a,b. Severe degree of epiphyseal compression from conservative splinting of neonate. X-rays of 2½-year-old male splinted at 5 months. The epiphysis is eccentrically reduced and there are epiphyseal and metaphyseal changes. AP and lateral X-rays of left hip.

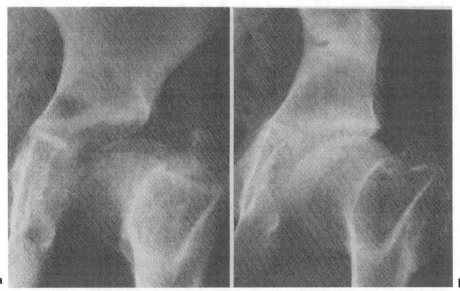

Fig. 5.34a,b. Late deformity of proximal third of femur associated with 5 cm of shortening. Same patient as in Fig. 5.33, now 12 years old. **a** Deformity involving coxa plana and short femoral neck with high greater trochanter. **b** Salvage surgery involving pelvic osteotomy to stabilise anterolateral subluxation and distal transplantation of greater trochanter.

decided to perform a pelvic osteotomy and transpose his greater trochanter, in an attempt to stabilise his hip joint. This major surgery was successful and he now walks without a limp, his latest X-rays being seen in Fig. 5.34.

It has been pointed out previously that while the femoral head remains cartilaginous, that is before the appearance of the proximal femoral epiphysis, it is susceptible to any mechanical compression caused by splinting when there is an incarcerated limbus. Such compression is transmitted through the cartilaginous head to act directly upon the proximal epiphyseal growth plate area. Kalamchi and MacEwen (1980) recognised that damage to the proximal femoral physis was not uncommon, as an iatrogenic complication following the treatment of CDH in this age group. They believed the insult to be vascular in nature and that the age of the patient at the commencement of treatment reflected the pattern and degree of deformity.

Thus it must be recognised that the bony components of the hip joint are more vulnerable to compression within the first 6 months of life, when there has been a pre-natal development and incarceration of the limbus. Fortunately many of these cases have a negative Ortolani test and are not picked up in the screening at birth and in the first 6 months of

life, but if the examiner is expert enough to detect any limitation of abduction and above-knee shortening, and elects to splint the child, there is a risk of permanent damage to the proximal femoral epiphysis and physis. This leads to permanent deformation and interference with proximal femoral growth. In such cases, elective treatment should be delayed until the infant is at least 10 months old, and if there is evidence of persistent displacement at this stage, then she is a candidate for infantile management.

David Trevor stated in 1967,

> Conservative treatment has had a long trial; it has not produced the goods. Its era is slowly passing and will be replaced eventually by the routine operative treatment of congenital dislocation of the hip. Satisfactory results in a much larger percentage of patients should be obtained and with a much shorter duration of treatment than by purely conservative measures.

Summary

1) All CDH at birth and during the first year of life can be and should be diagnosed clinically, but not all suspect cases turn out to be genuine.

2) X-rays and other forms of investigation are not always helpful and may be misleading until the appearance of the proximal femoral epiphysis.

3) The majority of babies born with CDH have hips in which the capsular ligaments are simply stretched by familial or hormonal joint laxity and mechanical derangement. They usually recover spontaneously.

4) The minority of babies born with CDH have an infolding of the stretched posterior capsule of the hip, and this can form an impediment to concentric reduction of the femoral head, making the diagnosis difficult due to the absence of a clear-cut Ortolani sign.

5) In this minority, early diagnosis might lead to early splinting and result in iatrogenic deformity, for as in talipes equinovarus (see Fig. 5.35) the bony components in the first 6–10 months of life are more susceptible to mechanical compression than the soft tissue impediments to reduction.

6) Post-natal development influences the response to management. Until the appearance of the proximal femoral epiphysis, the structure and blood supply of the femoral head is very susceptible to compression.

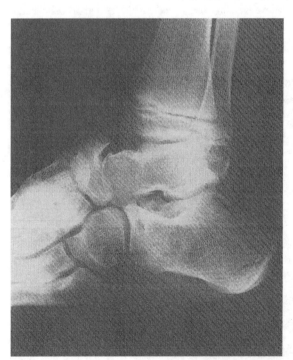

Fig. 5.35. Flat-topped talus in talipes, treated by wedged plaster at 3–6 months. The cartilaginous talus is more susceptible to mechanical forces than the soft tissue contractures.

References

Andren L, Von Rosen S (1958) The diagnosis of dislocation of the hip in newborns and the primary results of immediate treatment. Acta Radiol 49: 89

Andren L (1962) Pelvic instability in newborns. Acta Radiol [Suppl] 212

Barlow TG (1962) Early diagnosis and treatment of congenital dislocation of the hip. J Bone Joint Surg 44B: 292

Barlow TG (1966) Congenital dislocation of the hip in the newborn. Proc Soc Med 59: 1103

Bennet G, Catford J, Wilkinson JA (1982) The incidence of, and results of screening for congenital dislocation of the hip; Southampton 1965 to 1978. J Bone Joint Surg 64B(2): 243

Bertol P, MacNicol MF, Mitchell GP (1982) Radiographic features of neonatal congenital dislocation of the hip. J Bone Joint Surg 64B(2): 176

Bobath K (1966) Motor deficiency in patients with cerebral palsy. Clinics in Dev. Med. No. 23. Spastic International Medical Publications in association with William Heinemann, London

Browne D (1936) Congenital deformities of mechanical origin. Proc R Soc Med 29: 1409

Caffey J, Ames R, Silverman WA, Ryder CT, Hough G (1956) Contradiction of the congenital dysplasia—Pre-dislocation hypothesis of congenital dislocation of the hip through a study of the normal variation in acetabular angles at successive periods in infancy. Paediatrics 17: 632

Carter CO, Wilkinson JA (1964) Genetic and environmental factors in the aetiology of congenital dislocation of the hip. Clin Orthop 33: 119

Chapple CC, Davidson TD (1941) A study of the relationship between foetal position and certain congenital deformities. J Paediatr 18: 483

Chiari K (1953) Ergebnisse der Frühestbehandlung der angeborenen Huftgelenksverrenkung. Arch Orthop Unfall Chir 45: 644

Drachman DB, Coulombre AJ (1962) Experimental clubfoot and arthrogryphosis in multiplex congenita. Lancet 2: 523–526

Dunn P (1971) Congenital dislocation of the hips and congenital renal anomalies. Arch Dis Child 46: 878

Dunn P (1976) Perinatal observations on the aetiology of congenital dislocation of the hip. Clin Orthop 119: 11

Faber A (1937) Erbbiologische Untersuchungen über die Anlage zur angeborenen Huftverrenkung: Eine Röntgenologische-erbklinische Studie. Thieme, Stuttgart

Fredensborg N (1977) Congenital dislocation of the hip. Results of early diagnosis and treatment in Malmö. Int Orthop (SICOT) 1: 101–105

Hart V (1948) Congenital dysplasia of the hip joint and sequelae. Charles E. Thomas, Illinois

Hilgenreiner H (1925) On the early diagnosis and treatment of congenital dislocation of the hip. Med Klin 21(1): 385

Hippocrates The genuine works of Hippocrates. Translated from the Greek by Francis Adams, London (1849)

Howorth B (1963) The etiology of congenital dislocation of the hip. Clin Orthop 29:164–179

Hulbert KF (1950) Congenital torticollis. J Bone Joint Surg 32B(1): 50

James JIP (1970) The aetiology of scoliosis. J Bone Joint Surg 52B(3): 410

Jones D (1977) An assessment of the value of examination of the hip in the newborn. J Bone Joint Surg 59B: 318–322

Kalamchi A, MacEwen GD (1980) Avascular necrosis following treatment of congenital dislocation of the hip. J Bone Joint Surg 62A(6): 876–888

Le Damany P (1914) Congenital luxation of the hip. Am J Orthop Surg 11(4): 541

Lloyd-Roberts GC, Pilcher MF (1965) Structural idiopathic scoliosis in infancy. A study of the natural history of 100 patients. J Bone Joint Surg 47B(3): 520

Lloyd-Roberts GC, Swann M (1966) Pitfalls in the management of congenital dislocation of the hip. J Bone Joint Surg 48B: 666

Lorenz A (1895) Über die unblutige Behandlung angeborener Hüftverrenkung mittels der functionellen Belastungsmethode Zentralbl Chir 22: 761

MacKenzie IG (1972) Congenital dislocation of the hip: the development of a regional service. J Bone Joint Surg 54B: 18

McKeown T, Record RG (1951) Lancet 1: 192

Mitchell GP (1972) Problems in the early diagnosis and management of congenital dislocation of the hip. J Bone Joint Surg 54B(1): 4–17

Moraki A (1973) Die offene Reposition der angeborenen Huftluxation beim Säugling (German translation from Greek). Griech Operat Orthop Traumatol, Vol 24, No 2, Athens

Noble TC, Pullan CR, Craft AW, Leonard NA (1978) Difficulties in diagnosing and managing congenital dislocation of the hip. Br Med J 2: 260

Ortolani M (1948) La lussazione congenita dell'anca: Nuovi criteri diagnostici e profilattico-correttivi. Cappelli, Bologna

Ortolani M (1978) Detecting the dislocated hip. Correspondence in The Lancet, 4th March

Owen R (1968) Early diagnosis of the congenitally unstable hip. J Bone Joint Surg 50B(3): 453

Palmen K (1961) Preluxation of the hip joint. Acta Paediatr 50, Supplement 129

Pavlik A (1958) Die funktionelle Behandlungsmethode mittels Riemenbügel als Prinzip der konservativen Hüftgelenksverrenkungen der Säuglinge. Z Orthop 89: 341

Perkins G (1928) Signs by which to diagnose congenital dislocation of the hip. Lancet 1: 648

Place MJ, Parkin DM, Fitton JM (1978) Effectiveness of neonatal screening for congenital dislocation of the hip. Lancet 2: 249–250

Putti V (1929) Early treatment of congenital dislocation of the hip. J Bone Joint Surg 11: 798–809

Putti V (1933) Early treatment of congenital dislocation of the hip. J Bone Joint Surg 15: 16–21

Putti V (1935) Anatomia della lussazione congenita dell'anca. Cappelli, Bologna

Record RG, Edwards JH (1958) Environmental influence related to the aetiology of congenital dislocation of the hip. Br J Prev Soc Med 12(1): 8

Roser W (1879) quoted by K. Palmen (1961) Preluxation of the hip joint. Acta Paediatr 50, Supplement 129

Salter RB, Kostuick J, Dallas S (1969) Avascular necrosis of the femoral head as a complication of treatment for congenital dislocation of the hip in young children. A clinical and experimental investigation. Can J Surg 12: 44–61

Seddon HJ (1962) Dislocation of the hip. Editorial and Annotations, J Bone Joint Surg 44B(2): 255–256

Severin E (1941) Congenital dislocation of the hip joint. Late results of closed reduction. Acta Chir Scand 134, Suppl 63

Sharrard WJW, Grosfield I (1968) The management of deformity and paralysis of the foot in myelomeningocele. J Bone Joint Surg 50B(3): 456–465

Suzuki R (1979) Complications of the treatment of C.D.H. by the Pavlik harness. Int Orthop (SICOT) 3: 77–79

Tonnis D (1982) Congenital hip dislocation—Avascular necrosis. Theime–Stratton, New York Stuttgart

Trevor D (1957) Treatment of congenital dislocation of the hip. Editorial and Annotations, J Bone Joint Surg 39B(4): 611–613

Von Rosen S (1962) Diagnosis and treatment of congenital dislocationof the hip in the newborn. J Bone Joint Surg 44B: 284

Von Rosen S (1968) Further experience with congenital dislocation of the hip in the newborn. J Bone Joint Surg 50B: 538

Weinberg H, Pogrund H (1980) Effect of pelvic inclination on the pathogenesis of congenital hip dislocation. Isr J Med Sci 16: 229

Weissman SL, Toric G, Kermosh O (1961) Intertrochanteric osteotomy in fixed paralytic obliquity of the pelvis. J Bone Joint Surg 43A: 1135

Wilkinson JA (1972) A post-natal survey for congenital dislocation of the hip. J Bone Joint Surg 54B: 40

Wilkinson JA (1975) Failures in the management of congenital hip displacement in the newborn. Proc R Soc Med 68(8): 476–479

Williamson J (1972) Difficulties of early diagnosis and treatment of congenital dislocation of the hip in Northern Ireland. J Bone Joint Surg 54B(1): 13

Wynne-Davies R (1970) Acetabular dysplasia and familial joint laxity: two etiological factors in congenital dislocation of the hip. J Bone Joint Surg 52B(4): 704–716

Yamamuro T, Hama H, Takeda T, Skikata J, Sanada H (1977) Biochemical and hormonal factors in the etiology of congenital dislocation of the hip joint. Int Orthop (SICOT) 1: 231–236

Yamamuro T, Chene S-H (1975) A radiological study on the development of the hip joint in normal infants. J Jap Orthop Assoc 49: 421–439

6 Infantile Displacement of the Hip (10 Months to 3 Years)

Because I consider that the treatment of congenital dislocation of the hip is still a matter not merely of fundamental importance to Orthopaedic Surgeons, but also one on which the last word has not yet been spoken and which, therefore, it is opportune to discuss afresh.

Vittorio Putti (1933)

Our anatomical studies have revealed that CDH conforms to the general pattern of development affecting all congenital deformities in that the degree of deformation is maximal at birth. Then the pre-natal aetiological factors disappear and any subsequent development is dependent upon post-natal factors. Thus the clinical signs of hip displacement are maximal at birth and they should be detected by the trained orthopaedic examiner (Wilkinson 1972).

Those who would have us believe that CDH is simply a degree of hip instability at birth which is easily detected clinically must have great difficulty in explaining why the diligent search for its presence has not been too successful. The most exhaustive efforts in screening for hip instability have failed to reduce the number of persistent cases of CDH throughout the country.

In Southampton, where the screening of newborn is performed by our paediatric colleagues, between 1965 and 1978 only 30% of persistent cases were picked up at birth. Another 30% were diagnosed before their first birthday, but of the residual 40% only half were diagnosed before they were 18 months old (Catford et al. 1982). David and his colleagues in 1983 had the same experience in Manchester. They performed the same retrospective study on a series of 56 children with persistent CDH. These were first diagnosed after the age of 1 year, at the time when Barlow was teaching his methods of early diagnosis and treatment in the same area.

David et al. found that 23% of their series had never been examined at birth and there were another 20% that had been examined but found to be normal. Then more than 50% of the series were missed at birth. Another 20% had been picked up at birth and treated, but had not been kept under observation after the neonatal period and their displacements had recurred. These workers found that the parents were the first to notice something wrong with their children at approximately 11 months.

Parental Symptoms

David and his colleagues found that 18% of the patients had first-degree relatives affected. This is difficult to understand for it might be thought that a family incidence would have made the parents more aware of the dangers. Perhaps they had been over-reassured, inadvertently, of the unlikelihood of a second occurrence (see "Familial Risk", Chap. 4). Sixty-four per cent had been taken to health care professionals, but the diagnosis was missed or the child was not referred to hospital. In half of these the opportunity for diagnosis was missed either on more than one occasion, or by more than one professional. The study revealed the serious delay between the first parental symptoms of a dislocated hip and the eventual diagnosis, and the authors listed the more common complaints, including crawling difficulties, falling to one side, stamping and falling, and discomfort when legs were abducted such as sitting astride the mother's knee or when changing the napkin. The most frequent symptoms include limping in 55% and a short leg in 35% of cases. Previously Vittorio Putti in 1929, recorded:

> The loving eye of a mother does not miss even the slight evidence of asymmetry or abnormality. If you ask the mother what are her reasons for suspecting the deformity usually she will not answer precisely, she merely noticed some little asymmetry, something unusual in the shape of the outline or the attitude of one limb. One limb seems to be shorter than the other. One of the feet turns outward in separating the lower limbs. She saw or felt that one went less easily than the other. She observed that one limb was held in a certain degree of flexion or that if she tried to correct this flexion the child cried. It is just such small signs that makes one suspect a dislocation and which should induce one to have an X-ray examination.

He concluded that to improve the results of treatment of CDH, one must lower the age limit for beginning treatment, but to render this possible it is necessary for parents to learn to bring their children for medical examination early and for the doctor to be able to diagnose in time!

Although it may be understandable to overlook some cases of CDH within the first 2 months of life, it is a matter of concern that so many present symptomatically after the first birthday. Opportunities for earlier diagnosis are missed because the hips are not examined. The deficiency lies, therefore, not with the lack of parental interest in preventing sickness and disability, as more than 90% of parents bring their children to welfare clinics for immunisation, but rather the lack of awareness, motivation, and application of skills among health professionals. Catford et al. (1982) argued from the Southampton data that children attending for immunisation during the first year of life run a higher risk from undiagnosed CDH than they do from catching severe whooping cough.

Clinical Signs

Caffey et al. (1956) believed that the diagnosis of CDH was made much too late to permit optimum therapeutic results and that this delay was due to a lack of conspicuous clinical signs or symptoms prior to standing and walking. Vernon Hart (1948) disagreed, believing that such clinical signs were always present if one was diligent enough to search for them. Perhaps the diagnostic delay is due to the low prevalence of CDH and the temptation to restrict screening to those infants at risk, such as first-born girls, breech births, or those with familial histories. In concentrating the screening efforts to those at risk, the 40% of infants that are not at risk are frequently missed and their diagnosis is sometimes delayed until the child is 2 or 3 years old.

Lorenz (1895) is quoted as saying that CDH children are in general not only beautiful, but also flourishing with health as compared to the children with coxitis, who were so seldom like this, and that a distinction could be made from their faces in the hospital waiting room. Hilgenreiner (1935) stated that the children who are carriers of CDH in general are exceptionally pretty female children, and Sir Denis Browne taught that the typical patient was a first-born girl, from a full-term pregnancy, who usually turned out to be "blonde, buxom and beautiful", but the deformity was sometimes found in underdeveloped brunettes and also in boys (personal communication).

Whenever there is a family history of CDH it must be recognised that the prevalence is at least 30 times greater than normal and one should always scrutinise such children both clinically and radiologically or follow them up until it is certain that the hips are normal.

Signs of Breech Malposition

After the first 10 months of life much of the evidence of pre-natal moulding has disappeared. Sometimes plagiocephaly can persist until the third year of life and occasionally torticollis and the planovalgus moulding of the foot might also persist. All these signs should stimulate the examiner to check the hip joints.

Signs of Unilateral CDH

As 70% of persistent cases are unilateral, these signs are found in the majority of cases. The normal leg highlights the abnormalities on the abnormal side and expedites the diagnosis even in children before they are walking, whereas the majority of bilateral displacements are not detected until later, when the children have developed their waddling gaits.

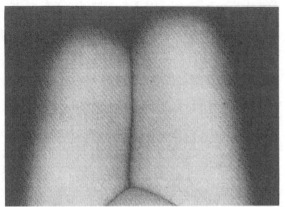

Fig. 6.1. Above-knee shortening in infant with unilateral, left CDH. With hips and knees flexed, the inequality becomes obvious from above.

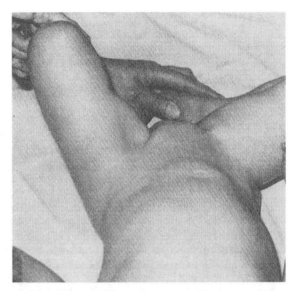

Fig. 6.2. Limitation of abduction due to adductor and anterior capsular contractures. Note the hollow in the adductor region—the sign of Joachimisthl.

Above-Knee Shortening. This is always present when compared to the normal leg and it is often associated with unequal folds in the perineum and adductor aspect of the thigh. These folds tend to deepen and become more prominent within the first year of life; as in new-born, the above-knee shortening in infantile cases can always be revealed by flexing both hips and knees to 90°. Such a posture often aggravates the displacement of the femoral head, making the inequality more apparent, as seen in Fig. 6.1.

Leg Posture. There may be an excess of lateral rotation of the thigh, which is due either to the displacement of the head of the femur out of the socket or to the degree of femoral retroversion that might persist at this time. The displaced hip is frequently abducted and flexed. There is often a poverty of movement in the affected leg and the child tends to hold the hip flexed and relatively immobile.

Limitation of Abduction. This is the most constant sign in infant displacement, but it is sometimes absent in cases where there is an extreme degree of familial joint laxity. Again it is better to demonstrate with the infant supine and the hips and knees being flexed 90°. The feet are held together and the knees are allowed to fall laterally into abduction to their full extent. On the affected side there is a resistance to further abduction at 50°–60°; the test is demonstrated in Fig. 6.2. The limitation of abduction can also be demonstrated with the child in the prone position. The inequality is usually apparent and the outer aspect of the affected leg appears to rise higher on the trunk than the normal side due to a prominence of the displaced greater trochanter.

This loss of movement is partly due to adductor muscle guarding, but it is also caused by contracture of the medial aspect of the capsule of the hip joint and the adductor tendons themselves. If the child is anaesthetised, the muscles relax to improve the range of abduction and this can be further increased by adductor tenotomy.

Hip Instability. At this age the Ortolani sign is usually negative, but it can persist in children with a marked degree of familial joint laxity, sometimes until the second or third year of life. Even in those cases when the Ortolani sign is negative, hip instability can be demonstrated by telescoping. The thigh is flexed to the vertical position and is held in the palm of the hand while the pelvis is fixed with the opposite hand. Instability can be detected by first pressing downward along the shaft of the femur and then lifting the thigh. This is probably one of the hardest signs to demonstrate in orthopaedics and it calls for much experience to detect abnormality.

Flattening of the Buttock. When the infant is in the prone position the buttock on the side of displacement appears flattened compared to the normal. This can be more easily appreciated by palpating with the flat of the palm.

Standing Posture. At this age children begin to stand, holding onto a chair, and one can observe their posture. If there is true shortening in one limb it is usual for the child to compensate by standing on the toes of the foot, holding the latter in equinus, but when the shortening is associated with hip instability the child flexes the opposite knee in order to bring the affected foot flat on the ground (Lloyd-Roberts and Swann 1966). Weight-bearing appears to aggravate the signs of leg shortening, making the inequality of skin creases more apparent.

Signs of Bilateral CDH

The diagnosis in such cases is far more difficult, as compared to unilateral displacements, because there is not a good limb for comparison to show up the inequality of leg length and the unequal skin creases; but when these children are looked upon as a whole, there appears to be a shortening of the legs compared to the trunk and if they are not too overfed the classical perineal gap is to be seen. Perkins (1928) stated that a normal child lying supine on a couch had the lateral outlines of the trunk and legs with a profile resembling that of an adult male, whereas the child with CDH has an outline approximating that of an adult female.

Raised Greater Trochanters. This can be appreciated by placing the examiner's thumbs on the anterior superior iliac spines and his index fingers on the greater trochanters (Fig. 6.3). It is necessary to learn the normal relationship of these two bony prominences in order to appreciate differences on one or both sides. The measurement can be taken with the child standing or supine, but the sign is not confined to CDH as it is also present in cases of congenital coxa vara. With experience this is an easier sign to elicit than the mapping out of Nelaton's line, as the latter involves probing for the ischeal tuberosity, which might be difficult in a plump child.

Limitation of Abduction. When both hips are dislocated, it is difficult to be sure whether limitation is abnormal, but at this age both hips should abduct sufficiently to allow the lateral aspect of the thighs to approximate the surface of the examination couch. Limitation of more than 40° must be very suspicious, especially when it is unequal. It should be remembered however that the sign may be absent in the presence of familial joint laxity even when both hips are displaced. As in unilateral CDH, it is sometimes better to perform the sign with the child lying prone with both hips extended.

Gait. At this age a waddling gait with frequent falls is sometimes a feature that more frequently amuses parents than alerts them to the fear of hip displacement. This might account for the delay in parental concern, as they only become worried when the habit persists. Lloyd-Roberts and Swann (1966) pointed out that the advent of a limp is often delayed for 4–6 months following the commencement of independent gait. When walking begins, balance is poor and there may be a considerable delay before the true Trendelenburg gait develops, "for this is an acquired skill of some complexity". This fact may also account for the delay in the diagnosis of bilateral cases, sometimes into the third year of life.

Radiological Signs

Soon after Professor William Conrad Roentgen discovered the diagnostic use of X-rays in 1895, Zenker in 1897 was thought to be the first to publish the first radiological evidence of congenital hip joint subluxation in a 3-year-old child (according to Wiberg, quoted by Hart in 1948). In 1900 Bade first recorded that the healthy side of unilateral dislocation showed hypoplasia of the roof of the acetabulum in 25% of X-rays, and John Ridlon (1906) confirmed this finding.

Dr Edward Shenton published his book *Disease in Bone and Its Detection by the X-rays* in 1911, in which he expressed the view that the careful surgeon never omitted to examine a young person with X-rays when CDH was suspected, as sometimes the clinical evidence was so obscure that ordinary methods failed to detect its presence. He described his diagnostic line which persisted intact in all positions of the joint:

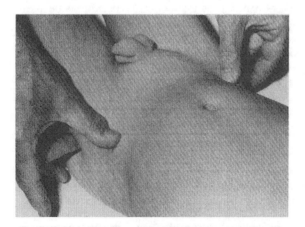

Fig. 6.3. Clinical assessment of height of greater trochanters. One should be able to appreciate any inequality and even bilateral displacement if the distance between the span of the thumb (on the ASIS) and finger (on the greater trochanter) is decreased.

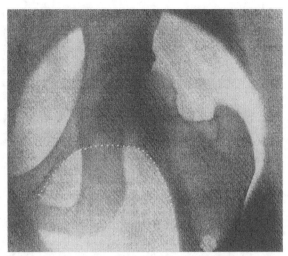

Fig. 6.4. Dr Shenton's original line (taken, with permission, from his book: Macmillan, London, 1911) "The line remained an unbroken arch formed by the top of the obturator foramen and the inner side of the femoral neck."

Tonnis (1976) confirmed the original observation made by Palmen (1961) that standard measurements of acetabular index could vary according to the rotation of the pelvis from side to side or in a sagittal plane, and described an index for the lateral rotation of the pelvis by dividing the diameter of the obturator foramen of the right side by that of the left side. He also evaluated the degree of inclination in the sagittal plane by measuring the angle between the symphysis and the os ischium. These are valuable methods of standardising X-rays before comparing the mean value of the normal acetabular index. He pointed out that this could not be measured after the age of 10 or 12 years and recommended the centre-edge angle of Wiberg (1933) for older children.

Diagnostic Features of Normal Hip Joints in Infants

Following the appearance of the proximal femoral epiphyses, the main feature of the normal radiological appearance is the positioning of these two growth centres within the circumference of the acetabula.

the line remained an unbroken arch formed by the top of the obturator foramen and the inner side of the femoral neck. Imagination must connect these two lines before a perfect arch is formed at a glance. X-rays will show that this line is a reality and not solely imaginative [as seen in Fig. 6.4].

Modern day clinical research involving the radiological screening of children with hip disease is dependent upon the standardisation of instruction with regard to obtaining standard views of the hip joints. In Southampton these standards are based on the conditions laid down in *Positioning in Radiography* (Clark 1980). In this manual the instruction for an anteroposterior film of the pelvis and both hips involves the patient lying in a supine position with the pelvis parallel to the film. Both feet are placed in a neutral position, preferably with the soles of the feet at right angles to the couch. The centre for both hips is the mid-line point, approximately 2 in. below the level of the anterior superior iliac spines and 1 in. above the upper border of the symphysis pubis. Lateral views are taken with the patients supine, the hips and knees being flexed by rotating the limbs laterally, through approximately 60°, with the thighs abducted to bring the soles of the feet into apposition. The limbs may be steadied by sponges and sandbags under the thighs. This position of the patient is aptly described as the "frog position" and the film is centred between the two hip joints.

The x-rays confirm the diagnosis, but the normal radiographic appearance of the pelvis and hip joints in very young children is not well known. It is as well, therefore, to have some simple guide by which one can tell at a glance whether the head of the femur is in its normal place [see Fig. 6.5]. Draw a horizontal line joining the innermost part of the ilium at the Y-shaped cartilage of the acetabulum. The bony nucleus of the head of the femur, as seen in the radiogram, should be below this line. Draw a vertical line from the anterior inferior spine (which is the prominent outer lower angle of the ilium as seen on the radiogram), cutting the horizontal line at right angles. The bony nucleus of the head of the femur should be internal to this line. These two lines will show whether the head of the femur is further up or further out than it should be. I have studied this in numerous x-rays of normal pelves of children under the age of 4, and I have never seen the bony nucleus of the head of the femur above the horizontal line, although occasionally the vertical line may just cut into it. These two lines enable one to gauge whether a reduction is complete, and also point out the minor degrees of subluxation which are so common (Perkins 1928).

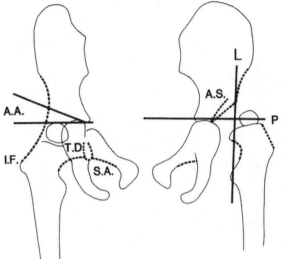

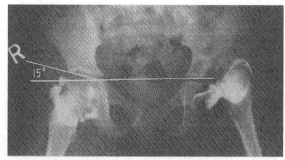

Fig. 6.6. Hilgenreiner's angle. Unilateral CDH with normal contralateral acetabular angle at 2 years, within the 1st standard deviation. (Wilkinson and Carter 1960, with permission)

Fig. 6.5. Measurements performed on standard X-ray. *S.A.*, Shenton's arc or line; *P.L.*, Perkins' parallel and vertical lines; *T.D.*, tear-drop; *A.A.*, acetabular angle; *I.F.*, ileofemoral line; *A.S.*, acetabular slope.

Kohler (1929) was the first to describe the "tear-drop" which is a feature on the floor of the normal acetabulum, the medial line being the outline of the pelvic wall and the lateral line being the anterior rim of the acetabulum. The tear-drop is absent in congenital displacement, and is often V-shaped or broadened in cases of residual subluxation. When the roof of the acetabulum appears bilabial, the medial dome-shaped curve represents the roof of the socket, whereas the lower straight line is the front edge of the acetabulum (Monk 1983). Shenton's arc has already been mentioned, but there is an equally important lateral iliofemoral line which is unbroken in concentrically reduced hip joints, whether the hip be extended, abducted or adducted, or flexed and abducted in the Lorenz position, as seen in Fig. 6.5. Hilgenreiner (1925) described a horizontal line between the two Y-cartilages, and also the angle between it and the line of the acetabular roof (see Fig. 6.6). This acetabular angle was used by Faber (1937), who published figures for normal children at birth, 2¾ months, and 12 months of age. Severin (1941) used the same measurement to assess dysplasia of the hip, and later Caffey et al. (1956) recorded the measurement at birth, 6 months, and 12 months. Massie and Howorth (1950) gave normal standards from birth to adult life, but unfortunately did not distinguish between the two sexes. Wilkinson and Carter (1960) measured 146 radiographs of normal girls and 128 of boys and obtained standards from 6 months to 4 years in both sexes. The highest angle found in undisplaced hips during

this age was 31°; figures above this indicated a degree of mechanical dysplasia secondary to subluxation. Tonnis (1976) repeated such measurement and found that his standard deviations concurred with the previous figures.

Diagnostic Features of CDH in Infants

Putti (1929) pointed out that radiological surveys revealed subluxations to be more common than dislocations. But whereas dislocations were more easily diagnosed and therefore treated earlier, subluxations did not become evident until later in life when normally every chance of a radical cure had gone. He described his triad of characteristic X-ray signs of hip displacement, which included:

1) The absence or diminished size of the proximal femoral epiphysis on the dislocated side. This sign is only applicable in unilateral dislocations and only after 6 months of life.
2) The top of the femur is some distance from the floor of the acetabulum and is higher than normal.
3) The roof of the acetabulum is sloping. However, this important sign is difficult to estimate because the divergence from the normal is small.

Modern radiological signs can be divided into four main groups:

Primary Deformities of the Pelvis. CDH is always associated with a lateral rotation of the affected side of the pelvis including the acetabulum, but these primary bony deformities can also be seen in the absence of displacement, as they are caused by the lateral rotation breech malposition. The iliac crest appears wider or narrower than normal and the obturator foramen is more open compared to the opposite side. Lateral rotation of the acetabulum produces an apparent dysplasia which increases the acetabular angle. There is also an enlargement of the pubic and ischial bones.

Signs of Dislocation. It usually appears that the proximal femoral epiphysis has been displaced both laterally and proximally, leaving a vacant acetabulum, yet in some cases of persistent subluxation, it may be difficult to appreciate the degree of displacement. One is then dependent upon a break in Shenton's line, or in the lateral iliofemoral line. With regard to Perkins' lines, the proximal epiphysis usually occupies the upper and outer quadrant when the hip is completely displaced, but in cases of subluxation it sometimes lies lateral to the vertical line but on the horizontal line or even below it. Displacement is never present when the epiphysis lies within the lower and inner quadrant. The femur is usually rotated laterally, producing an apparent coxa valga with a prominent lesser trochanter and bowing of the shaft.

Hypoplasia of Enchondral Ossification. The proximal femoral epiphysis is either absent or smaller than normal and sometimes its development may be irregular. This is due to a hypoplasia, or a delay of enchondral ossification in the femoral head. When the epiphysis is absent, its appearance may be delayed up to several months or occasionally 1 or 2 years. This is more relevant in unilateral displacements. There is also a hypoplasia of the acetabular roof due to a delay of enchondral ossification in the secondary centres of the acetabular rim. Delayed closure of the ischiopubic ramus is apparent compared to the opposite side in unilateral cases, but this is a feature of the general hypoplasia of the affected side of the pelvis.

Secondary Effects of Hip Displacement. Kohler's teardrop is absent in complete displacements, yet it may be present but distorted in subluxations. This is due to the disappearance of the lateral line or the anterior wall of the acetabulum, and also a thickening of the medial wall or the base of the acetabulum making the depth of the acetabulum appear inadequate. Biglow in 1844 described "the rising of the bottom of the socket" (quoted by Hart 1948) which seems to result from the absence of pressure. Then there is a notch above the outer margin of the acetabulum (MacKenzie 1972) which makes the latter more prominent when compared to the normal side in unilateral cases. The appearance may well be due to a pressure effect of the distorted limbus, or to the high attachment of the superior capsule of the joint.

Arthrography of the Hip Joint

Surgeons who are familiar with the intricate features of arthrography appear to be constantly aware of the importance of soft tissue deformation and the dangers of eccentric reduction in the management of CDH, whereas those who shun its significance rarely go out of their way to explore and deal with soft tissue impediments at the time of reduction.

Historical Review. The first attempt to demonstrate the soft tissue features of the hip joint was made by Gocht (1908) when he injected air into a post-mortem specimen and produced beautiful arthrographic studies. Dorach and Goldhamer in 1925 repeated these post-mortem studies by injecting a solution of potassium iodide intra-articularly. They identified the limbus and the zona orbicularis.

The first clinical studies were performed by Sievers and Bronner in 1927, according to Severin (1941). They injected iodopin into infant hip joints in their clinical studies of CDH and described the features of the capsule and limbus, and were the first to demonstrate its incarceration between the femoral head and acetabulum. Ortolani (1948) claimed that Putti (1937) was the first to start the study of the infant hip with contrast medium, but that he became so familiar with the clinical and functional study of the normal and the dislocated hip that he thought it of little practical use to continue the study. A diagrammatic representation of his findings is shown in Fig. 6.7. Ortolani himself used the technique to differentiate between preluxations, subluxations and dislocations, but came to the conclusion that it was not a useful investigation in the early stages of pre-dislocation, and used in preference his "snapping sign" to differentiate between the dysplastic hip which would benefit from conservative treatment and that which required surgery. In the latter he used arthrography to determine which type of treatment would be best. At the same time Ortolani quoted Faber (1938) who showed that 1-month-old babies with a radiological dysplasia of the hip often appeared to have a normal cartilaginous acetabulum, as demonstrated in Fig. 6.8. Faber laid down the following conditions for a normal articulation:

1) The tip of the limbus must come down in contact with a straight line drawn between the Y-cartilages.

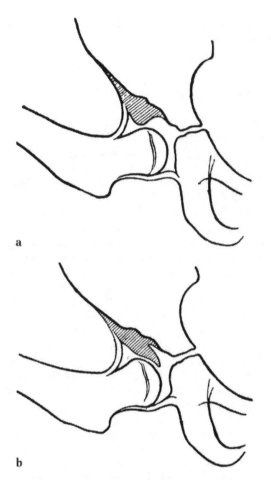

Fig. 6.7a,b. Putti's diagrams representing soft tissue obstacles to reduction. (Hart 1948, with permission)

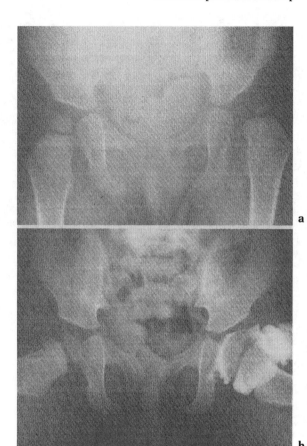

Fig. 6.9a,b. Normal arthrogram. **a** Apparent subluxation of left hip at 1 year. **b** After 3 weeks of vertical traction the hip remained stable and arthrography revealed a normal left hip according to the criteria laid down by Faber.

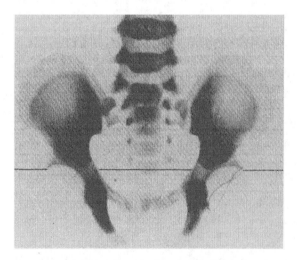

Fig. 6.8. Faber's new-born pelvis. The left acetabular edge has been painted with aluminium bronze. (Hart 1948, with permission)

2) The free edge of the cotyloid fibro-cartilage must clasp a good half of the head.

3) There must be no accumulation of contrasting substance between the head and the centre of the acetabulum.

Le Veuf (1947, 1948) became the master of arthrography in CDH and after a long experience involving many hundreds of patients he claimed that he was able to differentiate between subluxation and luxation, as demonstrated in Putti's diagram (see Fig. 6.7). Although he believed that subluxation and luxation had their origins in a common ground, "since both malformations may co-exist in one subject or may appear alternately in the course of hereditary transmission of the disease", he was quite adamant that from an initial stage, subluxation and luxation developed individually toward essentially different anatomical conditions, and that a subluxation never became a luxation post-natally. He began arthrography in 1935 and related the appearances to the surgical anatomy, claiming that this confirmation prevented him from falling into the trap that many other unwary investigators succumb to. In subluxations, the limbus was forced upward and outward towards the iliac fossa, whereas in luxations the limbus was forced downward and inward towards the acetabulum.

Yet there were many other differences affecting both soft tissue and bony components of the hip in these two conditions. In subluxations the capsule never appeared to be interposed between the femoral head and the acetabulum and the ligamentum teres was absent in about 50% of cases. There was an incongruity of the bony components, with the femoral head being larger than the acetabulum, which assumed an oval shape because of the atrophy of the roof. The femoral neck was valgus and anteversion developed early on. In luxations, however, the capsule was frequently interposed between the bony components, and the ligamentum teres was usually present. The acetabulum appeared normal, but its entrance was restricted by the limbus both superiorly and inferiorly. The femoral head appeared normal, whereas valgus deformity of the neck and anteversion of the femur only appeared late on in the development of persistent displacements.

From his findings Le Veuf came to the conclusion that the two arthrographic features indicating surgical intervention were eccentricity of reduction and incongruity of the articular surfaces. "There must be no accumulation of the contrasting substance between the femoral head and the centre of the acetabulum." His studies also showed that the Lorenz position gave a far better reduction of the femoral head than the abduction and medial rotation recommended by Putti. Failure to obtain concentricity of reduction led to residual subluxation and osteochondritis of the femoral head.

Technique of Arthrography. This invasive investigation is a very difficult procedure to develop, and it takes a long time before competence is gained. It is more difficult to perform when the hip is dislocated and also when it is reduced and stable. In this series the investigation has been confined to patients at the end of traction reduction of the hip, when the femoral head is contained within the acetabulum but remains dislocatable. It is performed under general anaesthesia, using the simple technique of injecting at a point distal to the anterior superior iliac spine, at the level of the mid-inguinal point, located by the pulsation of the femoral artery. The reduced femoral head can be palpated between the sartorius and tensor fascia lata as the hip is being moved, and one can insert the needle post-

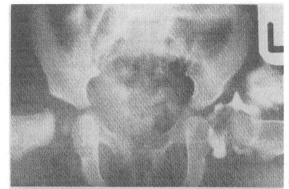
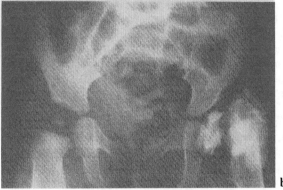

Fig. 6.10a,b. Arthrography in dislocatable hip. **a** Hip reduced revealing central pooling and inverted limbus. **b** Hip displaced revealing an incarcerated limbus and the conical shape of the cartilaginous femoral head.

eromedially into the joint cavity. If the hip is dislocatable, the femoral head can be displaced posteriorly, allowing the needle to enter the cavity without damaging the articular surface. Saline is first injected and the backflow confirms a successful penetration of the capsule. Then 5–10 ml Diodone (25% concentration) is introduced, before the withdrawal of the needle. When the hip is dislocatable, X-rays can be taken with the femoral head reduced and displaced, demonstrating in the former the eccentricity of reduction, and in the latter the soft tissue features of the capsule and limbus, as seen in Fig. 6.10.

Thus arthrography has been used in this present series to record the degree of soft tissue deformation of the affected joint, but sometimes it is necessary to confirm concentric reduction, also to differentiate between a stable reduction and an irreducible dislocation. Otherwise it has not helped in the management of routine cases, as the decision to proceed to arthrotomy depends upon the degree of instability of the hip at this time. In other words, if the reduction is unstable, it is assumed that this is due to an incarcerated limbus and this assumption is confirmed in more than 85% of cases. Yet arthrography has proved to be a great help and source of information in the retrospective study of our cases, especially in relating the size and shape of the cartilaginous femoral head to the outcome of treatment. Rarely it reveals an unsuspected septic arthritis of the hip joint, resulting in a partial or complete destruction of the femoral head. On one occasion it revealed a congenital coxa vara with an absence of the femoral head, in a previously unsuspected case, as shown in Fig. 6.11.

The technique is invasive and as such there is a threat of infection if it is not performed in the operating theatre with strict aseptic precautions. There is also the risk of morbidity due to damage sustained to the femoral head, especially when the investigation is left to the most junior and inexperienced member of the team. The margin of safety between perforating the capsule and the articular surface of the femoral head is small, being less if the hip is not dislocatable and does not contain excess synovial fluid. The injection also produces a temporary increase of the intra-articular pressure, and if this is not released by either aspirating or proceeding to arthrotomy, it could well embarrass the vascular supply to the femoral head and cause a mild form of avascular necrosis. Apart from these objections, arthrography is a very helpful investigation, especially in more difficult cases. In the words of Sir Harry Platt (1953), "a closer acquaintance with the detailed anatomy of congenital dislocation of the hips is derived from arthrographic studies, proving what Guilleminet and his associates (1952) have wisely said that each congenital dislocation has its own special morphology".

Computed Tomography in CDH

As the hip is a multi-axial joint variably situated on the pelvis, displacement of the femoral head out of the acetabulum may take place in a number of directions. Orthodox anteroposterior X-rays usually reveal any displacement in a coronal plane (superolateral), whereas anterior or posterior displacements and also rotational displacements remain cryptic. True lateral views of the acetabulum are difficult to acquire in infants, but Chuinard (1978) has developed the technique in older children and this has helped in the full assessment of the direction and degree of residual displacement.

Conventional tomography is not always available and when taken in an axial plane it involves excessive radiation. It is claimed that the use of stereophotogrammetry, in order to measure acetabular

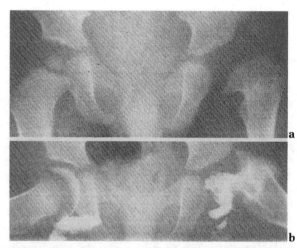

Fig. 6.11a,b. Unsuspected congenital coxa vara presenting clinically as infant CDH. **a** X-ray suggesting left CDH. **b** Arthrogram revealing a very small femoral head contained in restricted acetabulum. (By kind permission of Mr John Myles)

and femoral anteversion, is a superior technique. It involves less radiation and enables one to see the entire acetabulum and proximal femur as one image, from which to calculate the appropriate angle (Weintroub et al. 1981). They claim to have found acetabular anteversion from 0° to 30°, and femoral torsion ranging from 10° of retroversion to 80° of anteversion. Such refined techniques are not universally available and they call for a dedicated radiological team.

Thus it is hoped that computerised axial tomography will provide a non-invasive and helpful source of information, but early reports remain fragmentary and the technique is still to be developed to its full potential. There is no doubt that it is a foolproof method of measuring femoral anteversion (Weiner et al. 1978). It allows a visual portrayal of the cervical axis superimposed on the diacondylar axis, for direct goniometric measurement of the anteversion angle. Clinically this can only be performed with any degree of accuracy after the age of 2 years, when ossification has occurred in the femoral epiphyses and diaphyses. At that stage the maximal readings recorded are 30°–40° (Weiner and Cook 1980). Unfortunately these techniques involve high radiation dosages with present tomography machines, but this will probably improve in the future.

There is no doubt that computed tomography reveals the depth of the acetabulum and any degree of incongruity or subluxation of the femoral head, although according to present reports only posterior subluxation has been visualised, as seen in Fig. 6.12. Measurement of acetabular orientation is diffi-

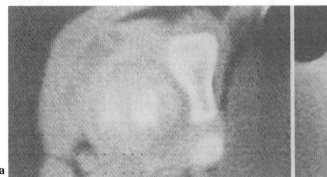
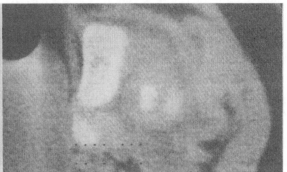

a b

Fig. 6.12a,b. Computed tomography, left CDH (infant). The left capital epiphysis and greater trochanter are hypoplastic and displaced posteriorly. There appears to be a true thickening of the iliac portion of the acetabulum.

cult, as the various levels cannot be related to pelvic orientation. To date, the measurements have been confined to the plane of the image rather than to the anatomical orientation. Earlier machines were dependent upon the ossification of the pubic bones and did not reveal any cartilaginous structures. Posterior subluxation of the femoral head out of the acetabulum appears to be associated with a hypoplasia of the anterior rim. This in itself will produce a false reading of acetabular anteversion, if the latter is dependent upon the plane of the acetabular rim related to the coronal plane of the anterior aspect of the pelvis, and not to the sagittal plane between the sacrum and pubic symphysis.

It is to be hoped that in future it might be possible to combine computed tomography with contrast arthrography and so reveal the relationship of the soft tissues to the bony components. This has already been attempted in the research on spinal conditions, but there have been no reports so far on CDH.

Computed tomography is a research implement which will reveal a great deal of information concerning the orientation and displacement of the components of the hip joint, but further work must be done, especially on normal hip structure, before we can assess accurately any abnormal deformation.

Nuclear Magnetic Resonance

It is only recently that nuclear magnetic resonance has been used in orthopaedics and it appears to visualise soft tissues, but bones do not produce an image, as seen in Fig. 6.13. Although experience in this technique is still in its infancy, it seems to have many advantages over computerised tomographic scanning. There is no hazard in its clinical use when

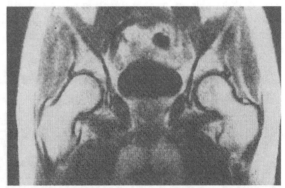

Fig. 6.13. Nuclear magnetic resonance. Routine scanning visualises soft tissues rather than bony components. This investigation appears to have greater potential than CT scanning in CDH.

applied by experts. Nuclear magnetic resonance is sensitive to blood flow and can demonstrate the intervertebral discs in relation to the neural canal.

The technique may prove to be superior to computerised tomography, as it can define soft tissue structures such as the limbus without any invasive arthrography. It may have the potential for a breakthrough in non-invasive visualisation of the hip joint, defining mainly its soft tissue structures—and it has been proved already that these have greater importance than the bony components (Steiner 1983).

Differential Diagnosis

There are a number of pitfalls in the diagnosis of infantile CDH for the unwary clinician and surgeon and there is not sufficient space to list them all.

There are, however, three conditions which continue to turn up in everyday surgery, not associated with generalised disease, and to be forewarned is to be forearmed. In addition there are two rarer conditions that mimic CDH clinically.

Septic Arthritis of the Hip Joint (Tom Smith Arthritis)

In 1874 Sir Thomas Smith recorded in the St. Bartholomew's Hospital Report a disease which he called "acute arthritis of infants". It usually occurred within the first year and was very dangerous to the life of the child, as well as intensely destructive to the articular ends of the long bones. A feature of the disease was that it rarely produced ankylosis of the joint, but left the child with the limb shortened by the loss of part of the articular end of some bone and with a weakened flail-like joint. Originally it was thought that most cases were due to

a mouth infection in breast-fed babies, which eventually led to a haematogenous osteomyelitis. This usually affected the hip joint, but sometimes the knees, shoulders, or elbows might also be involved and the disease can be multifocal.

Sometimes an abscess simply pointed and discharged onto the buttock, following which the infection settled, but not before destroying the proximal femoral epiphysis and physis. Such children could present later with the clinical signs mimicking congenital displacement of the hip, when all evidence of the infection had settled. The stigma was a healed, puckered scar on the buttock of the child, as taught by Sir Thomas Fairbank (1934). Even the radiological appearances could be deceptive, as seen in Fig. 6.14, as they mimicked a CDH with an absent proximal epiphysis and displacement of the proximal end of the femur. It is not unknown for the diagnosis to remain cryptic up to the time of arthrography, following attempted but failed reduction of a persistent dislocation.

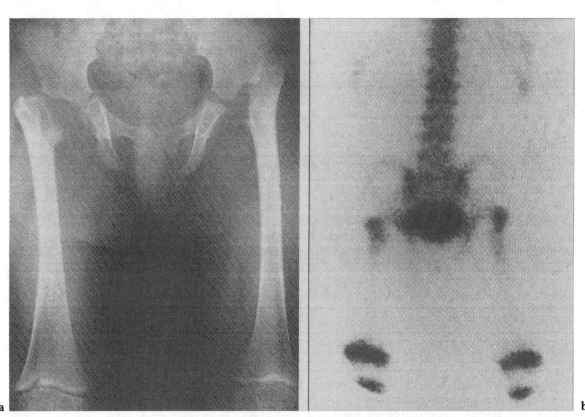

a   b

Fig. 6.14a,b. Septic arthritis of the hip joint. **a** X-ray of infant with multiple lesions affecting both hips and right knee. Note the right hip is destroyed, but not dislocated, as has occurred on the left side. **b** Bone scan of same patient revealing excessive bone activity in both hips and right distal femoral epiphysis, also showing displacement of left hip. N.B. Both hips were explored surgically. The right was totally destroyed, but the left femoral head was small and displaced and there was an inverted limbus. (By kind permission of General El-Geneidy)

In Egypt, today, there is still a very high prevalence of septic arthritis of the hip joint which is probably higher than the prevalence of congenital displacement in that country. Bone scanning has helped in the diagnosis, differentiating between a destroyed joint and a pathological dislocation. It is interesting to note that the latter more frequently affects the left hip and in these cases there may be lateral rotation of the left side of the pelvis and evidence of dysplasia of the bony components of the hip joint, suggesting that the infection might involve a previously congenitally displaced hip joint. The intra-articular structure of these joints also suggests an underlying congenital dysplasia, with infolding of the posterior capsule to form a limbus (similarly reported by Mitchell 1979). The advent of antibiotics has produced an even greater confusion, in that the child might well respond to such therapy and the septic arthritis settle, without even the formation of a sinus and scar to warn the clinician.

Traumatic Dislocation of the Hip Joint

Occasionally even a slight injury can displace the normal hip joint, especially in an infant girl with an excessive degree of familial joint laxity. The initial injury may be so trivial as to be missed, the child being brought a few days later to the clinic, because of pain and inability to walk. X-rays confirm a complete displacement of the femoral head, without any associated deformation of the pelvis and dysplasia of the acetabulum.

Reduction can usually be attained under general anaesthesia, and a short period of splinting in a plaster spica allows the joint to recover. Avascular necrosis is not common, but occasionally a slight degree of coxa magna develops within a few years (Offierski 1981).

Infantile Coxa Vara

Fairbank (1928) described two separate conditions, including a congenital group and another appearing in the infantile period. The congenital group is often associated with a bowing or shortening of the femur, whereas the infantile group usually have two clear lines through the neck of the femur in the form of an inverted V, as seen in Fig. 6.15. Fairbank thought this condition to be due to a developmental error in the femoral neck which led to progressive

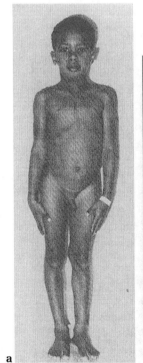
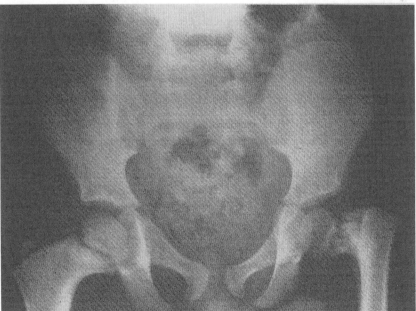

Fig. 6.15a,b. Congenital coxa vara, left hip. **a** Six-year-old boy with shorter left leg. Note pelvic obliquity and equinus foot to compensate for leg shortening. **b** Same patient. Bilateral coxa vara, mild degree of deformity on the right side, but severe on the left with inverted V-defect caused by stress fractures.

deformity during the early weight-bearing years. Subsequently, however, other writers have agreed that the cervical lesion is not congenital as it is not present at birth, but appears to be due to stress fractures occurring in infantile life.

Both groups mimic CDH in that there is a true shortening of the affected limb and a raised greater trochanter and limitation of abduction. The condition is commoner in girls (Elmslie 1913), two thirds of cases are unilateral, and the left hip is more commonly affected than the right. It is not unusual for the limp to appear soon after the child begins to walk, and in bilateral cases the waddling gait is not unlike that resulting from bilateral CDH. There may be above-knee shortening, amounting to 1 in. or more, and the distance between the greater trochanter and the anterior superior iliac spine is decreased accordingly. There is marked limitation of abduction and to a lesser extent medial rotation. The Trendelenburg sign is positive on the affected side. Radiologically, the presence of a clear line through the neck of the femur distal to the epiphyseal line, and sometimes two lines forming an inverted V enclosing between them a triangular piece of bone, is associated with a varus deformity of the femoral neck which is sometimes reduced to something

below a right angle. The acetabulum may be well formed, but it is sometimes shallow due to shelving of the upper margin. There may be a general asymmetry about the pelvis in unilateral cases.

Craniocleidodysostosis

This is a very rare congenital deformation which affects the pectoral girdle more commonly, but there is sometimes a congenital deficiency of the pubic symphysis with associated instability. This causes the child to walk with a waddling gait and often the Trendelenburg test is positive on both sides. Rarely, there is an associated congenital coxa vara which might also aggravate the instability of the hip joints, as seen in Fig. 6.16.

Ectopia Vesicae

This congenital malformation of the lower genitourinary system is associated with an absent pubic symphysis and lateral rotation of both acetabula. The children are usually bow-legged and walk with

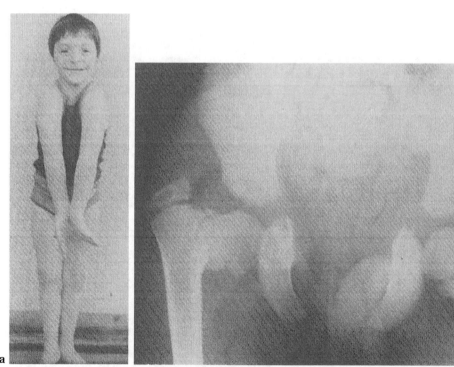

a   b

Fig. 6.16a,b. Craniocleidodysostosis. **a** Seven-year-old boy with absent clavicles able to approximate both shoulders anteriorly. **b** X-ray of pelvis reveals absent symphysis pubis. There is also bilateral congenital coxa vara which is sometimes associated with the condition.

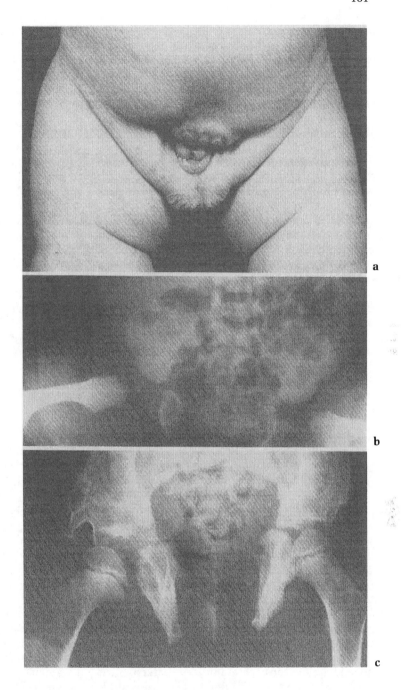

Fig. 6.17a–c. Ectopia vesicae. **a** Four-month-old boy with ectopic bladder. **b** X-ray reveals absent symphysis pubis and lateral rotation of both acetabula. The right hip is displaced. **c** Same patient 3 years later, following surgical reduction of right hip and both femoral and pelvic osteotomies.

a waddling gait. Very rarely, the condition can be associated with a CDH, which occurred in the patient seen in Fig. 6.17. The management of the combined pelvic and hip instability creates great difficulties, and it is fortunate the association of these two congenital problems is so rare. This might not be so, as ectopia vesicae is the commonest condition associated with a sagittal displacement or retroversion of the acetabula.

Surgical Management

The earliest attempt at treating young children with CDH involved heroic surgery, and Poggi (1888) is thought to be the first person to have performed a successful reduction, by retaining the femoral head in a deepened acetabulum. His techniques were later developed by Lorenz (1895), who used this opportunity to acquire an intimate knowledge of the surgical anatomy of the deformation. Later, the discovery of diagnostic radiology (Roentgen 1895) allowed a closer assessment of the bloodless methods of reduction, and encouraged people like Paci (1887) and Lorenz (1895) to develop their skilled methods of manipulative reduction and retention in plaster casts.

In 1900, Professor Lorenz issued the second edition of his volume on congenital luxations of the hip and in it he stated that 450 cases had been treated, with only three deaths from chloroform narcosis and another two who died from the manipulation! Davis (1903) pointed out the fact, little realised at that time, that there were very definite dangers in forcible manipulative reduction, listing a number of complications, including fractures of the femur and pelvis, peripheral nerve injuries, and even gangrene of the leg, in cases treated by Paci and Lorenz. Nevertheless Paci's method of circumduction, based on Bigelow's dictum on the reduction of traumatic dislocations, remained popular in Europe and America until 1950, and even later. It was described as a method of reduction by Bryan McFarland in Sir Thomas Fairbank's Birthday Volume (1956), and he considered the method to be simple and easy and the prognosis good in patients up to the age of about 18 months. Retrospective studies comparing closed manipulation with gradual abduction (Wilkinson and Carter 1960) revealed a very much higher incidence of epiphysitis or fragmentation in the more traumatic technique.

Meanwhile another school of management was advocating the reduction by the gentler forms of abduction. The founder was Professor Vittorio Putti who invented an apparatus that allowed a gradual degree of abduction in each limb separately. He claimed that 95% of CDH, in patients under the age of 12 months, reduced anatomically with a perfect functional result; his technique was published in 1929 and became accepted by many authorities. Later traction was added by various people, including Coonse (1933) and Keith (1935). The concept of atraumatic reduction, attained by gradually abducting the hips on a horizontal frame, was developed by Scott (1953) and he claimed that his technique reduced the prevalence of epiphysitis to less than 10%. The Wingfield frame had to be measured and made to fit each individual and this almost restricted its use to orthopaedic centres with appliance workshops. The management also called for specialised orthopaedic nursing care, as many of the children had to be sedated in the earlier stages and were often kept on the frames for periods up to 2 months. Sometimes it was necessary to apply cross-traction in order to bring the femoral head to

the level of the acetabulum to obtain satisfactory reduction. Even then, the majority of cases required surgery to attain concentric reduction, in order to prevent redislocation, as described by Somerville (1967).

Today, the lack of appliance fitters and the cost of providing tailored frames for each patient demands a simpler method. Also many infants are treated in the paediatric wards of general hospitals, where specialised orthopaedic nursing care is not always available. Thus it has become necessary to devise a simple technique of reduction on a standard frame for all infants. A vertical form of balanced traction has been developed similar to the Gallow's frame (Bryant 1880), but wide enough to allow gradual abduction of both legs. This method is not unique, as various forms of vertical traction have been used previously in the reduction of CDH. Traction without abduction was described by Salter et al. (1970), as pre-operative treatment. Maw et al. (1970) described a balanced vertical traction, including "guided abduction" with flexed knees to relax any hamstring contractures. Lloyd-Roberts (1971) also used fixed vertical traction on a hoop frame, but he found it necessary to apply cross-traction in order to attain satisfactory reduction.

Southampton Method of Reduction

In the treatment of CDH, success depends on the appreciation of a greater resistance by the soft tissues to mechanical compression, as compared to the bony components; the acetabular and femoral growth centres are extremely sensitive to compression and torsion. Transient and permanent deformities can result from over-enthusiastic efforts to reduce the displacement and also from the enforced splinting involved in conservative treatment.

In this series a simple form of balanced vertical traction has been used over the past 15 years, during which time 180 infants have been treated. The technique has been successful and it has produced a very low incidence of avascular necrosis, 3%–5%, as compared to other reported series (Massie 1951; Judet 1958).

The apparatus consists of a rigid metal frame, 135 cm wide and 90 cm high. It is clamped to the foot end of a cot and a stabilising strut is fixed to the footrail for added security, as demonstrated in Fig. 6.18. The horizontal and vertical bars are perforated by holes 10 cm apart, and large enough to accept the bolts of two adjustable pulleys. Two more pulleys remain fixed at a height 15 cm above the level of the cot. The head end of the cot is raised

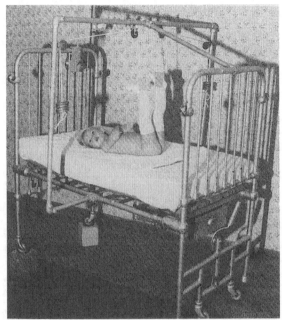

Fig. 6.18. The Alton vertical frame for reduction of infantile CDH (1). Child at the beginning of traction with legs vertical and sufficient but equal weights on both legs to raise the buttocks off the mattress. Note the head of the cot is elevated, so that voided urine runs downwards.

on 10-cm blocks, as this causes voided urine to run down and away from the child's buttocks and back.

Selection of Patients. Two thirds of our patients were diagnosed before their first birthday. Some, at birth, had failed to respond to simple treatment and others had not been splinted for reasons given in Chap. 5. These and other patients picked up in the neonatal period had their treatment delayed until the femoral epiphysis had appeared in the displaced hip joint. This gave the theoretical advantage of knowing that a mature blood supply had been established in the femoral head, and the practical gain that the resistance to mechanical compression was twice as strong as before the epiphysis had appeared. The epiphysis usually appeared before the tenth month, but its appearance was sometimes delayed until the eighteenth month.

On admission each child is examined very carefully to make sure there is no scar on the buttock or stigmata of spinal dysraphism in the sacral region. Any wasting of the calf or inequality of foot size is noted and an assessment of the degree of joint laxity in both upper and lower limbs is also made, as this affects the ease of reduction. X-rays are taken of the pelvis and hips to confirm the diagnosis and the presence of a femoral epiphysis, and chest films

rule out congenital heart disease and any other intrathoracic problems.

Southampton Management

The child is first examined under a general anaesthetic to assess whether the hip is reducible. If there is an adductor contracture a tenotomy is performed at this stage. There is no agreement on the efficacy of adductor tenotomy and even its advocates vary in their opinion as to when it is most effective. Tucker (1949) stated that when the hip adductors are tight, it would seem less dangerous to the circulation of the femoral head to lengthen them by tenotomy than to stretch them forcibly. MacKenzie et al. (1960) also stressed the benefits of adductor tenotomy and advised it routinely. If the procedure is to prevent any compression of the femoral head, tenotomy must be more effective at the very beginning of treatment. It is important to record whether the femoral head can be reduced before or after tenotomy and to assess whether or not reduction is unstable, as this will be compared to the degree of reduction at the end of traction. Most hips are reducible at this stage, but in some of the older children the joint may be irreducible at the beginning of traction. This does not contra-indicate the treatment, as the latter is aimed at stretching the anteromedial capsular contracture rather than reducing the dislocation. It attains eccentric reduction of the femoral head without compressing it in most cases, as shown in Fig. 6.19.

Skin traction is applied to each leg with the knees slightly flexed in order to relax the hamstrings. The child is placed on the frame while still under anaesthesia. Equal weights are added to apply balanced traction to each leg sufficient to raise the buttocks off the mattress ($\frac{1}{2}$–$1\frac{1}{2}$ kg each side). These weights are not varied during the period of traction. The most central pulleys are positioned in order to apply traction with the legs slightly abducted for the first 10 days. If a child has unilateral CDH the affected leg appears shorter at first, the heel being lower than on the normal side. It is not unusual to find the child is slightly irritable during the first week until the legs have equalised in length, after which she kicks and moves more freely and appears to be happier on traction.

During the next 10 days the central pulleys are moved laterally one hole every day, increasing the abduction of both legs by 10° on each occasion until finally reaching the lateral hole, when the legs are abducted 80° to the vertical on each side, as seen in Fig. 6.20.

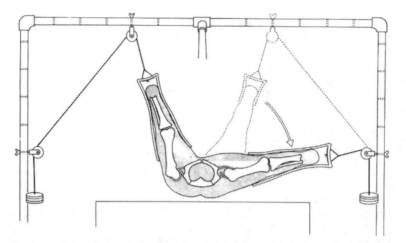

Fig. 6.19. Diagram of vertical traction (2). The anterior capsule on the right side is contracted at the beginning of traction, even following adductor tenotomy. It is stretched on the left side, at the end of the traction period, allowing eccentric reduction of the femoral head without compression.

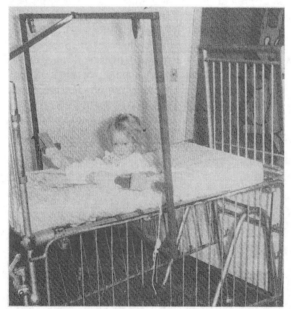

Fig. 6.20. The Alton vertical traction (3). After 10–14 days with the legs vertical, slow abduction of both legs is attained by moving the pulley laterally another hole every 2 days.

In this series the infants have tolerated the duration on the frame without any distress and sedation has never been necessary, as seen in Fig. 6.21. Infants with bilateral CDH are usually kept on traction for 4 weeks and the older patients for 6–8 weeks. It is not wise to use this technique in children over the age of 4 years, as their leg lengths are then likely to be more than 42 cm and for every 12 cm the foot is raised above the cardiac level the peripheral blood pressure drops by 10 mm Hg. The mean blood pressure in this age group is 77 mm Hg

at cardiac level (Haggarty et al. 1956) and this means that over the age of 4 years the peripheral circulation (arteriolar pressure) will fall to the danger level of near adequate perfusion (42 mm Hg) on vertical traction (Tanner 1946 and Prince, personal communication, 1980). Nicholson et al.

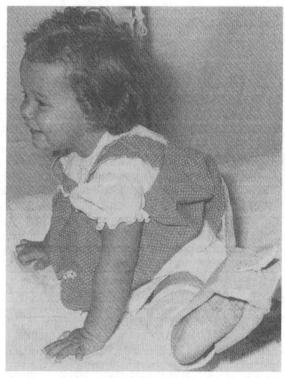

Fig. 6.21. Vertical traction (4). Another child appearing happier at the end of the traction period as her hip is reduced, but dislocatable.

(1955) suggested that hyperextension of the knee in children over 2 years of age might impede blood flow to the foot owing to the popliteus tendon constricting the main artery. If the knees are flexed to 10° while applying the traction strapping to the infant's legs, this will relax the popliteus and the hamstring muscles and prevent this mechanism from occurring. It has been suggested that abduction causes the infolding of a limbus and its secondary hypertrophy (Fergusson 1973), but this is not proven. In a small series of patients on vertical traction the legs were not abducted, but a limbus was found inverted in each joint treated. We did not proceed with this method, as the anterior capsular contracture was not stretched so effectively and limited abduction of the hip persisted in these children.

Results of Treatment. The series to date consists of 180 infants ranging from 10 months to 3 years of age including 230 CDH, as the series contained 50 bilateral cases. Of the infants, 60% were girls.

At the end of the traction period the child is examined under a second anaesthetic in order to assess the degree and stability of reduction. Arthrography can be performed at this stage to record the degree of soft tissue deformation. The results of traction can be separated into three groups:

1) Reduced, stable, and non-dislocatable hips accounted for 15% of the total. When there was doubt, arthrography confirmed concentric reduction. In cases where there had been no evidence of instability of the hips before traction and no previous history of a positive Ortolani sign, the infants are allowed to kick free at this stage but are followed up at regular intervals. Most of these cases turn out to be apparent displacements (Lloyd-Roberts and Swann 1966) and they undergo a spontaneous recovery as described in Chap. 5. If there is a history of previous instability, either at birth or at the time of the first examination under general anaesthesia, the stable hips are splinted by applying a Denis Browne harness for 6 months. The majority of these patients have persistent radiological acetabular dysplasia a year after reduction and come to pelvic osteotomy in order to stabilise the joints. At the time of this surgery, it is usual to explore the joint and find a small limbus incarcerated between the femoral head and acetabulum. It can be removed at this stage.

2) A second group of 83% of cases of CDH remain unstable or dislocatable at the end of traction. Arthrography in these cases reveals eccentric reduction of the femoral head with pooling of dye in the floor of the acetabulum and incarceration of the limbus.

It is necessary to proceed to posterior arthrotomy in this group, in order to excise the limbus and plicate the lax posterior capsule to obtain and stabilise the concentric reduction of the femoral head, before the child is placed in a Lorenz plaster. The hips are held above a right angle, but are not forcibly abducted to the neutral position. The child is discharged home in her plaster and it is retained for 2 months before being replaced with a Denis Browne harness which is maintained for a further 4 months. Six months following posterior arthrotomy the children are allowed to kick free and walk normally. In cases of bilateral hip displacement, bilateral arthrotomies are performed at the same time and their postoperative management is similar to that of unilateral CDH.

3) In a third, but very much smaller group, there were three failures to vertical traction, as the hips remained irreducible. The femoral heads could not be reduced into the acetabulum and were therefore not dislocatable. In such cases an excision of the soft tissue impediment through a posterior arthrotomy is a very difficult procedure, as there are often persistent capsular contractures. These patients are subjected to a formal surgical reduction through an anterolateral approach (Salter 1961). This exposes the anterosuperior aspect of the joint, allowing an extensive incision of the capsule to provide an unrestricted access to the acetabulum. In each case a large circumferential limbus has been found extending across the greater part of the acetabulum and creating a total obstruction to the reduction of the femoral head (Fig. 6.22). It is usual to find the ligamentum teres intact and it leads to a central hiatus in the limbus, under which lies the primary acetabulum which is usually of normal size and depth. Excision of the limbus allows a concentric reduction of the femoral head and the hips remain stable in the Lorenz plaster. Their post-operative care is as that described following posterior arthrotomy.

Posterior Arthrotomy. Only those infants whose hips remain dislocatable after their period of traction are prepared for posterior arthrotomy. The procedure is performed under the same anaesthetic, as it is not a major operation. The child is placed on her side with the affected hip upward, the leg being prepared and draped independently in order to allow free manipulation. The femoral head is reduced into the acetabulum and the hip is flexed, before a 4-cm incision is made extending obliquely upwards and backwards above the tip of the greater trochanter. The gluteus maximus is split along the line of its fibres and the posterior edge of the gluteus medius is then

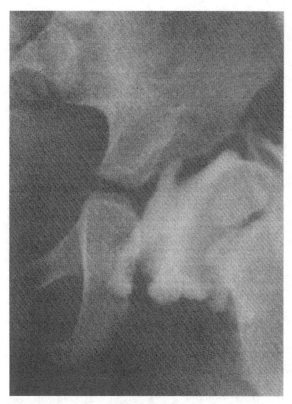

Fig. 6.22. Circumferential limbus, causing a complete obstruction to the femoral head, except for a small hiatus through which passes the ligamentum teres. Found in three infants' hips that failed to reduce on vertical traction. See anatomy in Fig. 7.4, p. 131.

identified. It is retracted upward to reveal the gluteus minimus and piriformis tendons. These two muscles are stripped from the underlying superior capsule and are again retracted superiorly and inferiorly respectively. A blunt hook is placed under the tip of the greater trochanter to pull it laterally and the rim of the acetabulum is then palpable deep to the posterior capsule between the gluteus medius and piriformis tendon, as seen in Fig. 6.23. An incision is made through the capsule parallel but lateral to the rim of the acetabulum. This allows synovial fluid to escape from the joint. The incision is extended superiorly and inferiorly in order to allow the retractors to be placed intra-articularly into the upper and lower limits of the joint. The blunt hook placed under the greater trochanter is then replaced to retract the lateral edge of the capsule. The medial edge is then incised at right angles to the previous incision down to the base of the limbus, revealed in the operative photograph (Fig. 6.24). Another blunt hook is introduced into the acetabulum in order to retract the limbus laterally out of the joint.

It can then be incised at its base, the incision being carried superiorly and inferiorly along its capsular attachment. Sometimes the limbus is adherent to the posterior articular surface and has to be gently lifted off by blunt dissection. It is excised under direct vision and is sometimes found to be in two layers, as shown in Fig. 6.25 (see also Fig. 5.30, p. 81). None of the excess capsule is excised, but it is reefed by placing deep polyethylene sutures well away from the incised edge. This stabilises the reduction of the femoral head. The wound is closed with a sub-cuticular Dexon suture.

If in bilateral CDH both hips are dislocatable, the first wound is sealed and then the child is turned onto the opposite side for the same operative procedure to be performed again on the other hip joint. Then the child is placed on a plaster frame in the supine position and both legs are placed in the Lorenz position, being flexed above a right angle and held in neutral rotation. Each thigh is allowed to fall into maximal abduction without force. Before the plaster is applied, both hips are tested to make sure they are reduced and it is important that this is done by the surgeon, who then applies the plaster, making sure that neither joint redislocates. Later, post-operative X-rays confirm that the reduction has been maintained. After 48 h the plaster is dry enough to make it waterproof and the child is then usually fit to be sent home.

The Lorenz Plaster. Adolf Lorenz (1918) was the first to appreciate that the splinting of a reduced hip was as important to the stabilisation of the articulation as was the previous reduction. In his original description of his method of retaining reduction by the application of a plaster spica, he advised an over-flexed and forcibly abducted position of the hips, in order that the femoral head should compress the floor of the socket. It was his way of deepening and widening the defective socket, before he adducted and extended the hip in serial plasters.

Our present appreciation of the susceptibility of the proximal femoral epiphysis to compression dissuades us from this forcible abduction, as forcing the hip in any direction might well be a cause of secondary osteochondritis. MacKenzie et al. (1960) condemned the Lorenz plaster on the evidence produced by Nicholson et al. (1954). Later Salter et al. (1969) reinforced this opinion with the results of animal experiments and advised the splintage of infants in the human position, in which the hips are flexed to more than a right angle, but only slightly abducted. In this series more than 200 infants with concentrically reduced hips have been splinted in Lorenz plasters and the prevalence of epiphyseal fragmentaion is lower than in any other series previously reported.

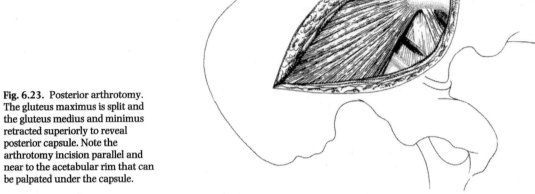

Fig. 6.23. Posterior arthrotomy. The gluteus maximus is split and the gluteus medius and minimus retracted superiorly to reveal posterior capsule. Note the arthrotomy incision parallel and near to the acetabular rim that can be palpated under the capsule.

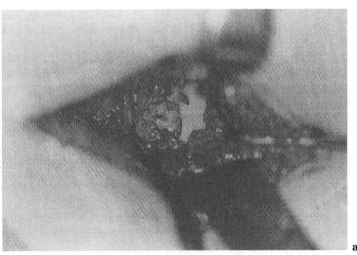

a

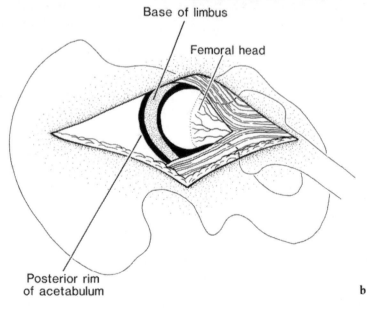

Base of limbus

Femoral head

Fig. 6.24a,b. Posterior arthrotomy. The posterior rim of the acetabulum is on the left separated from the peripheral base of the limbus, which lies between it and the femoral head. By applying lateral traction to the femur, the full extent of the limbus can be visualised. It can be detached superiorly and inferiorly with a sharp knife. After its excision the posterior capsule can be plicated by interrupted absorbable sutures, and the wound closed.

Posterior rim
of acetabulum

b

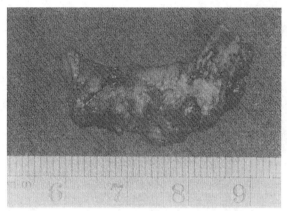

Fig. 6.25. Limbus, excised from dislocatable CDH through posterior arthrotomy. Its free edge is thin, but the attached edge is doubled.

It is believed that this clinical evidence proves the fallacy of the claim that the Lorenz position is a cause of epiphysitis. The position is demonstrated in Fig. 6.26.

The results of the series of animal experiments investigating femoral anteversion, reported in Chap. 2, revealed that the Lorenz position had great advantages as it corrected both femoral anteversion and retroversion, as compared to the Batchelor or Lange position of extension and medial rotation, which produced excessive anteversion. Thus there is no experimental evidence to support the claim by Tonnis (1982) that the Lorenz position is a cause of femoral anteversion, and this repudiation is strengthened by clinical practice (Wilkinson and Carter 1960).

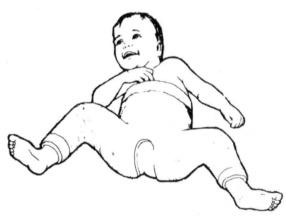

Fig. 6.26. The Lorenz plaster spica with both thighs flexed above a right angle, in approximately 60° of abduction and neutral rotation. Refer to Fig. 2.4 to understand its mechanism of correcting excessive femoral torsion.

Le Veuf (1947) demonstrated by arthrography that the Lorenz position gives a far better reduction than the position in abduction recommended by Putti, in other words, abduction and medial rotation. Beckett Howorth (1947) discovered that the greatest relaxation of the capsule is in the middle flexed position: "Thus the opening into the acetabulum should be largest with the hip flexed, and with a constricted capsule reduction should be more likely in some flexion than in extension. Furthermore the immobilisation of the hip in forced extension and medial rotation is likely to result in a temporary ischaemia by the torsion of the capsule, which may be followed by coxa plana."

Finally it is noted that those authorities who advocate the open reduction of the hip joint through an anterior or medial approach find it necessary to retain reduction by extending and medially rotating the hip joint, as this winds up the posterior capsule and stabilises the reduction (Ludloff 1913; Putti 1937; Fergusson 1973; Tonnis 1982).

Thus the belief that the Lorenz position is capable of producing avascular necrosis of the femoral head has not been confirmed in the present series. This might be due to the fact that the concentric reduction of the femoral head was obtained by the preliminary stretching of the anterior capsular contracture, followed by excision of the limbus before the hip was splinted in abduction and flexion in the Lorenz position. It may be that the combination of eccentric reduction and the Lorenz position is responsible for avascular necrosis. The very low prevalence of this complication in the present series is evidence to support this hypothesis.

When stability of the joint has been obtained within 6–8 weeks in a Lorenz plaster, it is safe enough to replace the latter with a Denis Browne abduction harness, seen in Fig. 6.27. This retains the 100° of flexion without forcibly abducting the legs, as the transverse metal bar is malleable and can be adjusted. The splint retains the neutral rotation without restricting rotational movements and this stimulates acetabular development and allows the vital abductors to develop rather than weaken and waste (Lloyd-Roberts and Swann 1966). Abduction splinting is maintained for 6 months before the child is allowed to kick free, extend her hips, and bear weight on the affected limb.

Alternative Methods

Le Veuf (1947) believed that concentric reduction of the femoral head could only be attained in CDH

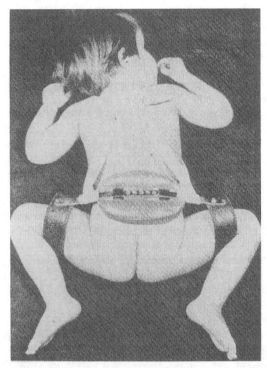

Fig. 6.27. Denis Browne abduction harness. It is essential that the cross-bar should be made of malleable stainless steel, so that it may be bowed not to forcibly abduct the hips. The cuffs should be rotated, so as to hold both thighs in the anchor position.

by surgery involving arthrotomy and excision of the soft tissue impediment, stating "it is a mistake to attempt bloodless reduction in such cases because it always fails". He had tried various forms of extra-articular techniques aimed at obtaining concentric reduction, including splintage, femoral osteotomy to correct the excessive anteversion, and also valgus osteotomy of the femur, but he found them all to fail and reverted to arthrotomy.

Severin (1941) believed otherwise and convinced himself and many of his contemporaries that the soft tissue barrier to concentric reduction in CDH could often be overcome by simply splinting the hip in abduction. He stated "an unsatisfactory condition immediately after the reduction with the limbus bent into the joint and signs of the head not reaching the acetabular floor, need not mean that the results of reduction will be poor". These conclusions were reached following the management of 330 infant patients with 454 congenital dislocations. He assessed them radiologically and found that 4.24 developed into normal hip joints, but another 7.14 had a moderate deformation. Eight per cent were dysplastic and 44% had residual subluxation. Thirteen per cent developed a secondary

acetabulum above the site of the primary socket and 17% redislocated. Influenced by Severin's teaching, MacKenzie et al. (1960) came to the conclusion that "closed reduction can give reasonably satisfactory and durable results in a fair proportion of cases", but they also had a 25% prevalence of avascular necrosis and a 15% failure rate in patients presenting before 3 years of age. More recently Vickers and Catterall (1980) advocated a 6-week trial of closed reduction in patients under 2 years of age, whose dislocations were previously reduced by vertical traction. By this method they found that 66% of the patients avoided open reduction, but that 20% developed evidence of avascular necrosis.

In this present series, it has been accepted from the outset of treatment that persistent displacement of the hip beyond the first 6 months of life is invariably due to the presence of a limbus (Somerville 1957). When the latter is large enough to prevent concentric reduction of the femoral head, it causes persistent instability following traction. The splinting of an eccentrically reduced hip is bound to lead to compression of the femoral head and acetabular roof with the risk of dire consequences. It is our experience with posterior arthrotomy that it is not possible to evert the limbus and gain concentric reduction of the femoral head. As it is an abnormal structure due to the infolding of the capsule and not a hypertrophy of the normal labrum, there is no reason for delaying its excision. Any attempt to evert and retain the limbus might well lead to further inversion, incarceration, and a recurrence of the eccentricity of reduction. At the beginning of the series, a clinical experiment was performed in bilateral CDH. At the end of vertical traction, when both hips were found to be dislocatable, only one was subjected to posterior arthrotomy. The more unstable hip was chosen, the other being reduced eccentrically and splinted in a Lorenz plaster. Eventually both hips usually came to pelvic osteotomy to correct the persistent acetabular dysplasia, and when operating upon the hip with the limbus, the joint was explored. The limbus was always found incarcerated in the joint and had to be excised in order to gain concentric reduction. Subsequent X-rays revealed a delay in the ossification of the femoral epiphysis on the side in which the limbus was retained until pelvic osteotomy, and the effects of compression persisted for many years, as shown in Fig. 6.28. Thus there was no evidence to support Severin's claim that the soft tissue barrier could be overcome by compression of the femoral head.

Ludloff in 1913 was one of the first to express dissatisfaction over the results of conservative management involving reduction by manipulation and

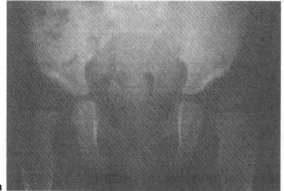

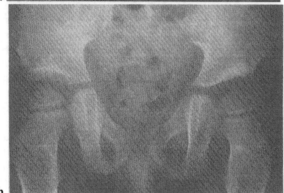

Fig. 6.28a,b. Bilateral infantile CDH. **a** Two years old, 1 year after reduction and excision of left limbus only. Note the hypoplasia of the right femoral epiphysis compared to the left. **b** Four years old, 2 years after bilateral pelvic osteotomy and excision of limbus on the right side. This epiphysis is still not developed as well as the left hip.

Lorenz plaster splinting, pointing out that even some early cases treated expertly failed to respond and redislocated once the plaster cast or splints were removed. His anatomical dissections revealed the variations from the normal structure in displaced hip joints. He came to the conclusion "that folding of the limbus and inter-position of the capsule are much more frequent than heretofore believed hindrances to reduction and retention, and are best eliminated by open operation". His paper contained one of the earliest references to the pathological limbus and its formation, which he held responsible for the failures of conservative treatment. He also described the contracture of the anterior capsule and believed that this was another cause of reluxation. This prompted him to advocate an antero-inferior approach to the intra-articular structures in order to release the anterior capsular contracture and excise the posterior limbus. Unfortunately surgery was in its infancy at that time and the results of such heroic attempts were complicated by infection, as well as an interference of the blood supply to the

femoral head. The disastrous outcome of many of these early attempts at surgical reduction caused his contemporaries to abandon this method of treatment and return to the more conservative methods.

Somerville and Scott (1957) revived Ludloff's work and confirmed his original findings, that the impediment to reduction was usually an infolded limbus which extended along the posterior and superior rim of the acetabulum. Somerville taught that it was only possible to remove this limbus through a restricted arthrotomy, when the hip joint was dislocatable. He approached the hip through an anterosuperior incision of the capsule instead of the antero-inferior incision described by Ludloff, and in so doing he managed to approach the posterior aspect of the joint over the summit of the displaced femoral head without having to divide the ligamentum teres. Unfortunately, he found that the hips were only stable in extension and medial rotation following this approach and applied his hip spicas in this position, as previously advocated by Ludloff (Somerville and Scott 1957; Batchelor 1959). Although Somerville believed that the limbus was a hypertrophied labrum, because of his failure to section it and identify its nature, it is opportune to pay him the acknowledgement that he deserves for reviving Ludloff's work and pioneering the indications for restricted arthrotomy and "limbusectomy". It is important that we in this country remember his teaching and perpetuate his practice. It is to be hoped that our North American and European colleagues acknowledge the importance of concentric reduction attained by excision of the limbus, and follow in our footsteps.

More recently, Fergusson (1973) expressed disenchantment concerning the pre-operative period of traction on a frame and held it responsible for the enlargement and inversion of the limbus. He also believed that there was ample evidence that the abducted or flexed position of the hip produced pathological changes in both the affected and normal joints due to pressure on the soft tissues. This led him to the conclusion that preliminary traction was unnecessary and he advocated a primary surgical reduction through the old Ludloff iliofemoral approach. His aim was to release the contractures of the anterior capsule and iliopsoas tendon, but he did not consider either the ligamentum teres or the limbus to be intra-articular obstacles to primary reduction. As Ludloff and Somerville discovered beforehand, Fergusson also found it necessary to splint the hip joint in extension, abduction, and medial rotation for at least 4 months postoperatively. Many have tried to emulate Fergusson's technique, but they have encountered recurrent instability post-operatively and some were forced to perform osteotomies to prevent the development of late residual subluxation (Tsuchiya and Yamanda 1978; Weinstein 1980).

Residual Bony Incongruity

Although it is acknowledged that concentric reduction of the displaced femoral head and containment by abduction splinting stimulates recovery of the acetabular and femoral dysplasia, there is an inherent incongruity (Platt 1953) which appears to become more indolent in its response to these factors in older children. The incongruity is partly due to the primary deformation of the bony components (see Chaps. 2 and 3) and also to post-natal development. After the period of splinting, in order to obtain full extension of the leg it is necessary for the hip to rotate 90° medially, so that the knee and foot point forward. The adoption of this new posture encourages both femoral and acetabular anteversion. Salter (1961) pointed out that such postural adaptation is greatest soon after birth, but gradually decreases thereafter. When there is any degree of laxity of the capsular ligaments, the torsion is not transmitted fully between the proximal end of the femur and the pelvis. Thus femoral anteversion develops, but the acetabulum may remain more retroverted in its primary position. This incongruous combination will tend to produce anterior subluxation as the hip extends, as seen in Fig. 6.29.

Southampton Management. Following the reduction of the CDH and the 6 months of abduction splinting, the 18-month-old infant is allowed to kick free, extending her hips and walking for the first time. After a further 6 months, the congruity and stability of the affected hip is assessed, when the infant is 2 years old. At that time there is usually evidence of persistent acetabular dysplasia and rarely subluxation of the femoral head, as seen in Figs. 6.30 and 6.31. Much of the dysplasia and subluxation might well be apparent, due to the persistent lateral rotation of the affected side of the pelvis. Realignment of the acetabulum and femur can be attained by osteotomy, either above or below the hip joint; whereas pelvic osteotomy increases the degree of acetabular anteversion to accommodate the normal degree of femoral anteversion, femoral osteotomy retroverts the femoral head to align it with the more retroverted acetabulum. Each procedure will result in bony congruity and stability of the hip joint, and subsequent remodelling of both bony components produces a similar degree of success, as seen in Fig. 6.31.

Pelvic (Innominate) Osteotomy. In his essay on the surgical treatment of CDH, Ernest Hey Groves (1928) was one of the first to use a triangular piece of bone from the iliac crest as a free bone-graft, in order to stabilise the dysplastic hip joint. In his technique of acetabuloplasty, he also included a skiagram, shown in Fig. 6.32, which must represent the first record of a pelvic osteotomy. It demonstrates a complete division of the pelvis above the acetabulum and the insertion of a triangular bone graft across the whole width of the pelvis, with lateral displacement of the acetabulum. In his essay, Hey Groves mentions the fact that he had been trying a new method, but it was too soon to speak of final results although they had been distinctly encouraging.

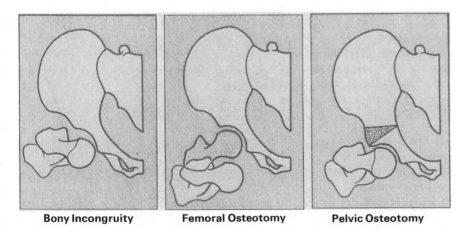

Bony Incongruity   Femoral Osteotomy   Pelvic Osteotomy

Fig. 6.29. Post-reduction infantile displacement. On extension of the hip and the development of femoral anteversion, the latter becomes incongruous with acetabular retroversion (see Fig. 3.20) and anterolateral subluxation occurs. This can be corrected surgically, either by femoral osteotomy or by pelvic osteotomy, each procedure producing bony congruity.

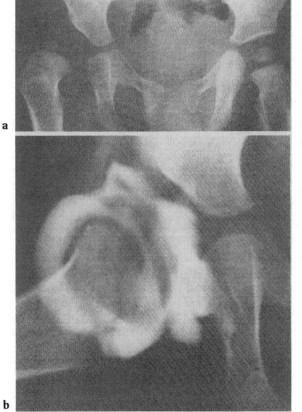

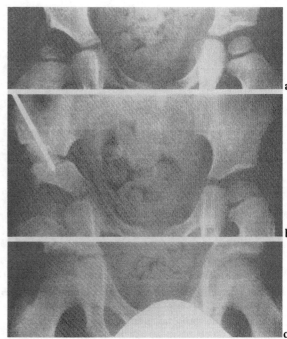

Fig. 6.31a–c. Infantile right CDH in the same boy, 1 year after reduction. a Persistent acetabular dysplasia, but no residual subluxation or epiphysitis. b Extra-articular pelvic osteotomy. c Ten years old, at 9-year follow-up. Grade 1 result—excellent.

Fig. 6.30a,b. Infantile right CDH. a Male, 10 months old. Left hip normal. b Right arthrogram—dislocatable hip after 3 weeks of vertical traction with eccentric reduction. Posterior arthrotomy and excision of limbus.

Salter (1961) developed the technique of acetabular reorientation and must be given the full credit for the development of the procedure which he calls "innominate osteotomy". His method reorientates the acetabulum anteriorly, laterally, and inferiorly, as he considers the primary deformity to be a laterally and superiorly placed socket. Salter uses innominate osteotomy as a technique of stabilising the reduction of a congenital displacement in children over the age of 18 months and frequently combines it with open reduction and capsulorrhaphy.

In Southampton, we have opted for a two-stage operative correction of infantile CDH, electing to attain concentric reduction of the displaced head at the age of 10 months, or later within the second or third year of life, and then correcting bony incongruity a year later. Our reasons for this two-stage procedure are based on the belief that the sooner concentric reduction is attained, the better for the future congruity of the articulation. It is very diffi-

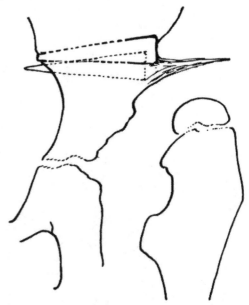

Fig. 6.32. Skiagram: First recorded impression of a pelvic osteotomy. (Hey Groves 1928, with permission)

cult to perform a pelvic osteotomy under 2 years of age, because of the "wafer thinness" of the pelvis, and one also encounters the risk of post-operative posterior subluxation of the femoral head if it is done while the femur is retroverted, in other words before the child is walking. Apart from this, it is felt the morbidity of both operative procedures is far less when staging the open reduction to precede the pelvic osteotomy compared to the combined procedure as advocated by Salter. Tonnis (1982) has recorded a similar experience in Germany, stating, "the studies of our material supported the view held in the literature that additional interventions at the time of open reduction of the dislocated femoral head result in an increased incidence of necrosis". On the other hand it was shown that an additional intervention, at 1–6 months following the open reduction, did not increase the incidence of necrosis. In Southampton we originally practised Salter's technique of open reduction, capsulorrhaphy, and pelvic osteotomy in infants presenting for the first time after their second birthday, but the outcome of their treatment was inferior and we have reverted to the two-stage procedure in all patients under the age of $3\frac{1}{2}$ years.

At the beginning of this series the operative technique of pelvic osteotomy was that described by Salter (1961) and I am indebted to his personal demonstration of this technique. Subsequently the operative procedure has been modified for two reasons: (1) the earlier reduction of the congenital displacement at 10–18 months has enabled one to restrict pelvic osteotomy to an extra-articular procedure, through a more limited approach; and (2) as the effects of decompression upon the femoral epiphysis have become more obvious, the operative procedure has been adapted to this principle at the time of reorientating the acetabulum. The technique of innominate osteotomy has been fully described by Salter (1961, 1983) and it is not intended to repeat the details fully; rather only my modifications will be described.

The incision used in this approach to the iliac crest has now levelled to a horizontal one, extending from the mid-inguinal point to the mid-iliac crest. It involves a subcutaneous dissection to reveal the iliac crest, but the scar is confined to the most modern "bikini area" and heals with minimal blemish when subcuticular absorbable sutures are used. Unfortunately, it usually means removing the transfixion pins through a separate incision at a later date. With regard to the techniques of decompressing the hip, Scaglietti and Calandriello (1962) emphasised that the extra-articular obstacles to an atraumatic reduction of the femoral head mainly involved contractures of the gluteus medius and iliopsoas and "such made it difficult to pull the head of the femur down to the level of the acetabulum". He advocated division of the psoas tendon and the origin of gluteus medius from the ilium to "reduce

later pressure on the capital epiphysis". Salter recommended psoas release, as a necessary procedure to reorientation of the acetabulum and his technique involved isolating the tendon above the rim of the acetabulum in order to divide it at this level. Originally in this series, it was found simpler to divide the iliopsoas tendon at its insertion into the lesser trochanter through a separate medial approach, but later it was easier to decompress by lowering the eventual height of the iliac crest. Now the upper third of the iliac crest is removed, and only part of it used as a graft to insert at the site of osteotomy. This means that at the end of the procedure, when the two halves of the iliac apophysis are sutured together, it is done without any tension, as seen in Fig. 6.33. Salter advocates the excision of a triangular graft from the anterior aspect of the pelvis, but when this is inserted at the site of osteotomy, it tends to increase the height of the iliac crest. By using the upper third of the ilium to provide the graft one produces a relative lengthening of the abductors and flexors and this removes any compression of the head of the femur (see Fig. 6.34).

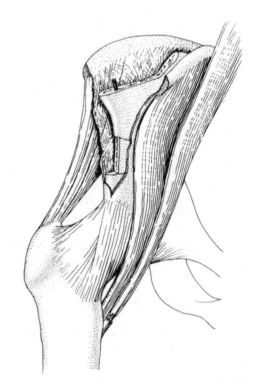

Fig. 6.33. Pelvic osteotomy. Excision of the upper third of the iliac crest, using only part of it for the osteotomy graft, lowers the final height of the crest and allows apposition of the two halves of the apophysis without any tension. Note the anterior displacement of the lower pelvic segment, the graft displacing it laterally.

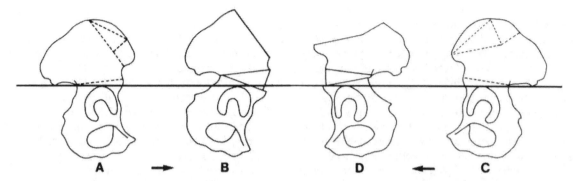

Fig. 6.34. Techniques of pelvic and innominate osteotomies. A→B Salter's method; D←C Wilkinson's method. When B and D are compared, the height of the crest is lower in D in relation to the acetabulum.

Thus, there is a relative lengthening of the gluteus medius and minimus, as well as the tensor fascia lata and iliopsoas muscles. The rectus femoris is also lengthened in front of the capsule of the hip joint by performing a Z-plasty, and this completes the decompression of the joint except for the adductor and hamstring muscles.

These important modifications have made it almost unknown for children to have any stiffness of their hips following pelvic osteotomy, and the long-term follow-up reveals little or no evidence of loss of epiphyseal height resulting from compression. The acetabulum is reorientated, by displacing the lower segment of the pelvis forward and laterally at the site of osteotomy, the assistant applying traction to the flexed hip and knee on the ipsilateral side. The insertion of the triangular graft, taken from the excised upper third of the iliac crest, holds the lower segment in its new position. Two transfixing wires are used now, including an anterior vertical wire and a posterior oblique wire, as in the early part of the series some of the wires extruded within the first 6 post-operative weeks with a loss of the displacement of the lower segment. This meant repeating the osteotomy.

Post-operatively, the child is kept in a one and a half hip spica extending on the operative side to below-the-knee level (see Fig. 6.35). Both hips are extended in abduction with slight medial rotation, and the knee is flexed on the side of surgery in order to relax the hamstrings and retain the degree of femoral rotation. The plaster is maintained for 6 weeks, during which time the child is allowed to go home. At the end of this period, the child is readmitted for removal of plaster and a week of hydrotherapy in order to provide the non-weight-bearing exercises to mobilise the hip. Within 6 weeks from surgery, the osteotomy is united and the child quickly regains a full range of movements, before being allowed to bear weight on the affected

leg. She is usually walking normally within 8 weeks from surgery. Four months from surgery, the pins are removed through a small stab incision made under general anaesthesia. This procedure can be performed on a day-patient basis.

The children are reviewed every year following surgery and this involves clinical and radiological assessment. After the age of 6 years, the serial assessments are extended to every 2 years until skeletal maturity is attained, in other words at puberty. If there is any radiological evidence of persistent or increasing instability in the serial X-rays during the follow-up period, a repeat pelvic osteotomy is performed (McEwen 1978).

Femoral Osteotomy. Although Le Damany (1908) had been the first to describe femoral ante-torsion as a dislocating factor in CDH, it was first recognised as a complication of treatment by Ludloff (1913). Later Badgeley (1949) believed it to be a primary fault in the aetiology of CDH, being responsible for an anterior displacement of the hip. His theories were elaborated by Somerville (1953), who advised

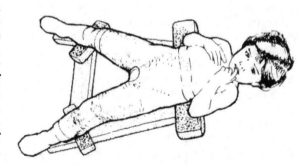

Fig. 6.35. Hip spica used following pelvic osteotomy. Max Harrison has pointed out the possibility of spontaneous dislocation of the opposite hip joint when a single spica is used (personal communication).

early correction within 4–6 weeks of reduction. Trevor (1957) advocated femoral osteotomy in order to restore the bony congruity and stabilisation of congenital dislocations. Subsequently the procedure has continued to be the most popular technique in many orthopaedic centres in Great Britain (Lloyd-Roberts and Swann 1966; Mitchell 1972; Vickers and Catterall 1980).

Femoral anteversion has been found to be an exceptional cause of failure in conservative treatment involving the use of a Lorenz plaster and Denis Browne harness to retain reduction (Wilkinson and Carter 1960). It has already been noted that those authorities who attain surgical concentric reduction through a medial, anterior, or anterolateral approach find it necessary to splint the child's limbs in the Batchelor or Lange position of extension and medial rotation, and appear to be concerned about the degree of femoral anteversion as a cause of residual subluxation. The experimental work in Chap. 2 explains these clinical observations, as Lorenz plasters appear capable of correcting excessive femoral anteversion and retroversion, whereas the internal or medial rotation splints persistently produce femoral anteversion. Other experiments in young puppies have shown that 60% of any surgically imposed femoral rotational deformity is lost within 2–3 months, due to remodelling by muscle activity (Schneider 1962). Fortunately this means that any over-correction of anteversion produced by surgical measures will disappear spontaneously.

More recently, computed tomography has produced an accurate measurement of femoral torsion as compared to clinical assessment and the results suggest that the problem has been over-estimated in the past (Weiner and Cook 1980). Lloyd-Roberts and Swann (1966) pointed out that the effects of lateral rotation femoral osteotomy can be neutralised by the patient simply standing and walking with the foot laterally rotated, but that this mechanism is overcome by adding a varus component to the femoral osteotomy. Subsequently Mitchell has shown that 20° of varus is equivalent to 1 cm of femoral shortening and this might explain the success of such a procedure in helping to decompress the hip joint. Recently Barnes (1980) has described premature partial closing of the proximal femoral epiphysis in Perthes disease, following femoral osteotomy and considers it to be due to an asymmetrical compression of the lateral part of the growth plate. He further suggests that femoral osteotomy might also be the final insult to an already precarious blood supply. Post-operative bone scans support this view, suggesting that femoral osteotomy is complicated by a relative ischaemia of the femoral head.

Mitchell (1980) believes that the removal of the plate and screws used in the internal fixation of femoral osteotomy might stimulate bone growth and be responsible for femoral lengthening and leg inequality, with its secondary aggravation of hip instability. His findings persuaded him to stop removing these metal implants. Finally the superficial scarring of the thigh resulting from vertical surgical incisions over the outer aspect of the upper third usually creates a major cosmetic blemish, as shown in Fig. 6.36. This is partly due to the fact that femoral osteotomy usually turns out to be a two-stage procedure involving the insertion and the removal of plate and screws at a later date, but it is also due to the vertical nature of the incision.

Thus, although femoral osteotomy like pelvic osteotomy restores the congruity of the bony components of the hip joint in CDH, by converting femoral anteversion into retroversion, as seen in Fig. 6.37, the evidence provided above strongly suggests that the femoral diaphysis should be considered a no-go area for the orthopaedic surgeon in this field of surgery, when there is a suitable alternative. As will be seen later, there are indications for femoral shortening in older patients with residual subluxation and dislocation, but in the younger age group pelvic osteotomy is the treatment of choice. It not only corrects the incongruity between the bony components of the hip joint, but also tends to decompress the articulation, whereas femoral osteotomy may compress it. The incision involved in pelvic osteotomy heals very well with minimal scarring, but even this can be hidden by the briefest bikini!

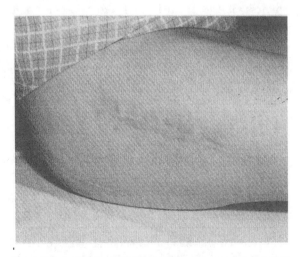

Fig. 6.36. Residual scar from femoral osteotomy, often keloid and ugly owing to its vertical position on the thigh.

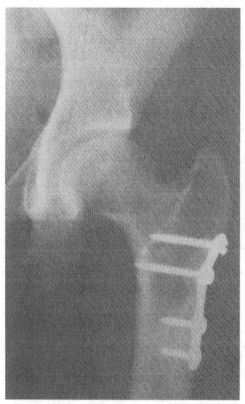

Fig. 6.37. Femoral osteotomy. The procedure has produced congruity and stability in this patient, with a loss of epiphyseal height and residual coxa plana.

Complications of Surgical Management

The failure of treatment in infantile CDH is manifested by three early complications, namely stiffness of the treated joint, redislocation, and avascular necrosis of the proximal femoral epiphysis, resulting in incongruity of the articular surfaces and residual subluxation.

Stiffness. Although this was not uncommon in patients treated conservatively (Wilkinson and Carter 1960) and has been reported in other surgical series, it was found that following the two-stage surgical treatment of CDH limited movements were relatively uncommon. After the first stage including posterior arthrotomy and abduction splinting for 6 months the infants were usually able to extend and adduct their legs fully within 2–3 months and there was no limitation of medial rotation. Subsequently the majority of these children walked and ran normally, and it was difficult to persuade some parents a year from the time of reduction that pelvic osteotomy was necessary, as the only indication was

the radiological appearance of the hip. In those cases where the displaced hip was irreducible at the end of traction and the child had to be subjected to a formal anterolateral open reduction, they sometimes developed a contracture of the abductor muscles during the 6 months of splinting. In one or two patients this persisted to a certain degree until the time of osteotomy, when any fixed degree of abduction was released by adequate excision of the upper third of the iliac crest, as previously advocated by Soutter (1914).

There has been little evidence of stiffness in any of our patients after the 6 weeks in a plaster spica, following pelvic osteotomy when concentric reduction of the hip has been obtained. Limitation of adduction and medial rotation producing an apparent lengthening of the affected leg is usually a sign of eccentric reduction. In such cases the child should be kept under close clinical and radiological observation as spontaneous recovery might not occur.

Redislocation. In the assessment of patients treated conservatively at Great Ormond Street (Wilkinson and Carter 1960), redislocation of the hip occurred early in the treatment in patients with persistent eccentric reduction combined with acetabular dysplasia. It occurred in 8 of the 107 patients with unilateral dislocation and 5 of the 84 bilateral dislocations, making a prevalence of almost 15% in the whole series.

In the present surgical management, when concentric reduction was obtained by surgery in all patients with unstable hips, it is not surprising to record that only two cases were known to redislocate. Both were girls with bilateral CDH, a family history and evidence of extreme degrees of familial joint laxity. On each ocasion the hips were stabilised by repeating the pelvic osteotomy and at the same time plicating the lax capsule, as shown in Fig. 6.38.

Avascular Necrosis.

Avascular necrosis of the femoral head is one of the most dreaded complications of the management of any congenital dislocation of the hip. Whereas many of the sequelae of delayed diagnosis or unsatisfactory results from conservative treatment are amenable to surgical correction, any major necrosis leaves adverse consequences throughout life. Surgical measures are then no longer capable of modifying the shape of the femoral head or influencing the damage done. The consequence is abnormal growth with early osteoarthritis, pain and disability. (Tonnis 1982)

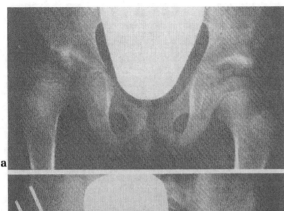

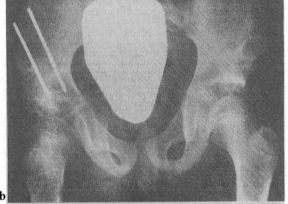

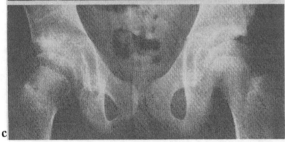

Fig. 6.38a–c. Bilateral infantile CDH. Failure of posterior arthrotomy and pelvic osteotomy salvaged by repeat pelvic osteotomy and plication of lax capsule. **a** One year after bilateral pelvic osteotomies. Residual subluxation of right hip. Grade 4. **b** Repeat right pelvic osteotomy and plication. **c** Seven years later. Right hip has been stabilised.

In the previous series treated conservatively (Wilkinson and Carter 1960), two degrees of fragmentation of the proximal femoral epiphysis were observed and described. There was a lesser form which constituted a transient, but punctate fragmentation in the pattern of density of the epiphysis. Similar changes have been described as a temporary vascular disturbance following the reduction of CDH (Salter et al. 1969; Bucholz and Ogden 1978). Yet a more severe degree of avascular necrosis was sometimes observed, producing a deformation of the femoral head and a permanent coxa plana. Occasionally it was associated with a thickening of the

neck of the femur, but otherwise there was little evidence of interference with metaphyseal bone growth. The severe changes were only observed in those hips reduced by manipulation under general anaesthesia. In retrospect, it is possible that there was little damage to the physis because the majority of patients were more than 18 months old, and there was a significant tendency for patients attending during the second year to do better than those attending earlier (Wilkinson and Carter 1960).

Avascular necrosis of the femoral head appearing after reduction of a CDH in young children was considered to be a preventable iatrogenic complication by Salter et al. in 1969. They also found that the femoral head was most vulnerable to the complication during the first 18 months of life, and especially in the first 6 months of life, when the femoral head is entirely cartilaginous. It affected nearly 30% of their children under the age of 18 months, particularly those in whom continuous traction was not applied before reduction. Scott (1953) believed that manipulative reduction was the main cause of severe osteochondritis and claimed to reduce these changes to less than 10% by frame reduction. Previously Tucker (1949) found that his research corrected the erroneous view that surgical division of the capsule necessarily impaired the circulation of the femoral head and suggested that splintage in abduction and lateral rotation might affect the posterolateral reticular vessels that were all-important in the vascular supply to the proximal femoral epiphysis.

In the present series, a mild degree of fragmentation with punctate changes in the epiphysis occurred in 12 hips following reduction. The changes first appeared in the X-ray taken a year from the time of arthrotomy, as similarly reported subsequently by Tonnis (1982). In six patients the changes were transient and disappeared soon after pelvic osteotomy. In two hips, a persistent coxa magna developed. In another two hips there was a subsequent partial loss in height of the femoral epiphysis, without any incongruity of the femoral head. The significance of such changes is not known at present, but they might have some unfavourable significance in view of the recent work in Perthes' disease (Hall 1980).

It is interesting to note that Somerville (1967) claimed to have no cases of osteochondritis, except for two delayed appearances in his patients. His series and the present series are the only two in which excision of the limbus has been performed routinely on dislocatable hips previously reduced by traction and controlled abduction. The management of each series is very similar, except that Somerville used a horizontal frame and later treated residual bone incongruity by femoral osteotomy. The common factor which is unique to both series is the early correction of eccentric reduction, through a restricted surgical approach, without any trial period of closed reduction and before the application of splints. The significance can be seen by comparing the very low incidence of avascular necrosis in both series, to that recorded in other series in which patients were not treated by routine surgery and were splinted in eccentric reduction; as for instance the 15%–30% reported by Salter et al. Joseph Truetta (1968) in his *Studies of the Development and Decay of the Human Frame* pointed out that continuous severe pressure affects growth, by interference with the circulation adjacent to the growing cartilage. This might well explain the dire effect of the incarcerated limbus in the eccentrically reduced femoral head in the management of CDH.

In the present series there were two patients who exhibited a mild degree of fragmentation before pelvic osteotomy, and subsequently developed a partial but deforming fragmentation of the epiphysis following pelvic osteotomy. Both developed a degree of coxa plana with minimal loss of femoral head congruity. The changes were sufficient to lower the results of treatment from Grade 1 to Grade 2. Thus

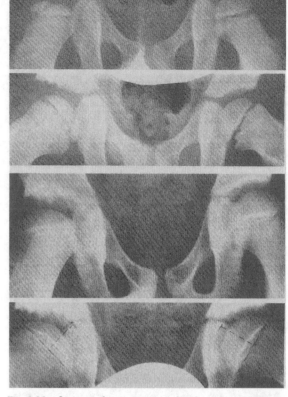

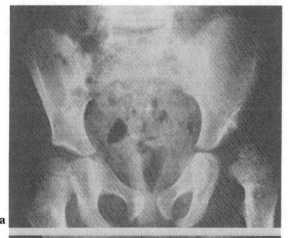

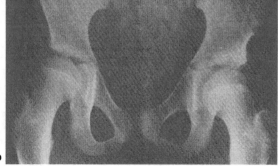

Fig. 6.39a–d. Avascular necrosis in infantile CDH. **a** *Mild degree*, 1 year after posterior arthrotomy and before pelvic osteotomy. **b** Eight years after pelvic osteotomy. No incongruity or loss of epiphyseal height, but slight coxa magna. **c** *Severe degree*, 1 year after pelvic osteotomy. **d** Five years after pelvic osteotomy. Coxa plana and loss of epiphyseal height = 1 cm.

the prevalence of permanent and severe fragmentation in this series is less than 2%, and this compares favourably to any other series. Such changes have not appeared since the technique of hip decompression has been included in the operative procedure of pelvic osteotomy, see Fig. 6.39.

Assessment of Results

Since 1966, a consecutive series of infants have been treated for persistent displacement of their hip joints at the Lord Mayor Treloar Orthopaedic Hospital, Alton, England. This personal series is made up of 180 patients to date, in which 230 persistent hip displacements have concluded their treatment. The series comprised 85% girls. Eighty were born before 1976 and treated before 1978. This means that there is a minimum follow-up period of 5 years since the termination of treatment, which is thought adequate for the assessment of the early results of treatment. The older members were treated in the earlier part of the series and have subsequently passed through puberty to reach skeletal maturity. Thus we are able to assess their final outcome.

In a similar series of patients treated conservatively, at the Hospital for Sick Children, Great Ormond Street, London, during the years 1948–1954, it was decided that the radiological results were far more critical than any clinical assessment (Wilkinson and Carter 1960). Five grades were proposed and these were very similar to those suggested by Wiberg in 1939 and Severin in 1941; they are shown in Fig. 6.40.

Grade 1. This hip appears to be almost normal. The acetabular roof is well developed, covering at least four fifths of the femoral head (Wiberg's C.E. angle equals 25° or more). There is no incongruity of the articular surfaces, and no loss of height in the epiphysis as measured from the midpoint of the epiphyseal line vertically to the acetabular roof (Hall 1981). Any residual stigmata of the previous displacement are trivial.

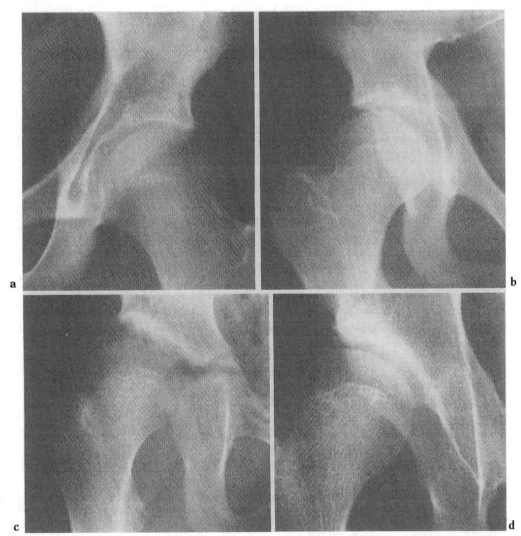

Fig. 6.40a–d. Long-term follow-up (10 years or more) in infant CDH treated by posterior arthrotomy and pelvic osteotomy. **a** Grade 1 result in 13-year-old girl. **b** Grade 2 result in 14-year-old girl. **c** Grade 3 result in 8-year-old girl. **d** Grade 4 result in same girl at 12 years. The last patient is an example of further subluxation during the pre-menstrual growth spurt. Such patients are now submitted to repeat pelvic osteotomy.

Grade 2. These hips resemble Grade 1, except there may be a partial failure of development in the acetabular roof, covering between two thirds and four fifths of the femoral head (Wiberg's C.E. angle equals 20°–25°). The articular surfaces are congruous, but sometimes there may be a slight loss of epiphyseal height associated with some minimal flattening of the femoral head, or even a minor degree of coxa magna from a mild form of epiphysitis; however there is no apparent subluxation.

Grade 3. In this group there is a moderately severe degree of acetabular dysplasia, with only half or two thirds of the femoral head being covered by the shallow roof (Wiberg's C.E. angle equals 10°–20°). Deformation of the femoral head is as listed in Group 2, but may be a little more severe; yet the congruity of the articular surfaces remains normal and Shenton's line is not broken. There may be a slight increase in the width of the medial joint space, but no further evidence of subluxation.

Grade 4. These cases reveal a definite residual subluxation, associated with a very shallow dysplastic acetabulum (Wiberg's C.E. angle is now negative). The instability is either due to a severe degree of genetic acetabular dysplasia, or a mechanical dysplasia secondary to a severe deformity of the femoral head resulting from fragmentation. There may also be a marked degree of coxa magna, or on the other hand, there can be a loss of epiphyseal height with some degree of coxa plana. The medial joint space may also be widened because of the residual instability, and Shenton's line is also broken, indicating a definite degree of residual subluxation.

Grade 5. This group contained hips that had redislocated, or the femoral head was contained in a false acetabulum. Yet there were no such results in our present series, treated surgically, to compare with these from conservative management.

These groups are readily recognised and the grading is very practical. Grades 1 and 2 are considered to be excellent and very good successful results. Grade 3 cases were originally thought to be on the borderline, but now they have been grouped with Grade 4 to be considered failures of surgical management, because of their bad prognosis. The majority of such patients have undergone salvage surgery, at a later date, in order to stabilise their hip joints. This usually involved a repeat pelvic osteotomy, the outcome of which is shown in Fig. 6.41. Although this will have stabilised the subluxating joints, their initial treatment has been considered a failure, as the results of delayed surgery have not been taken into consideration in this assessment.

Results. All the hips have been assessed separately in this series, and retrospectively there does not appear to be any significant difference between the results of unilateral and bilateral cases. The overall results are shown in Table 6.1.

Two girls were not subjected to arthrotomy because their hips were non-dislocatable at the end of traction, and a year later their hips appeared to be near normal; so it was decided not to subject them to pelvic osteotomy. One was unilateral and the other had bilateral displacements. The results were Grade 1 in the three hips. In the remainder of the series, 1 in 4 hips was stable by the end of traction and not subjected to posterior arthrotomy, but all came to pelvic osteotomy later on. In all displaced hips an incarcerated limbus was found, except in two that were not dislocatable at the end

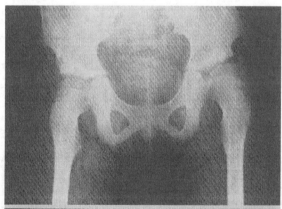

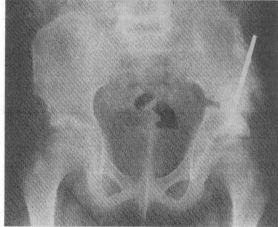

Fig. 6.41a,b. Late subluxation in pre-puberty phase. a Bilateral CDH. Left hip Grade 4, residual subluxation occurring at 10 years. Coxa magna due to persistent subluxation. b Same patient, left hip being stabilised by repeat pelvic osteotomy.

Table 6.1. Results comparing the outcome of conservative treatment in 1960, to the present surgical management

Treatment	Successful		Failure			Total no.
	1	2	3	4	5	
Conservative 1948–54	42	33	37	34	45	
		75		116		191
		39 per cent		61 per cent		hips
Surgical 1965–75	75	19	4	2		
		94		6		100
		94 per cent		6 per cent		hips

of traction and in which no limbus was found at pelvic osteotomy. Thus in all the 100 cases of CDH assessed, except for the three which escaped any surgery and the two that were non-dislocatable but not found to have a limbus at pelvic osteotomy, there was an incarcerated limbus in each joint; in other words, in 95% of cases.

In the initial part of the series, pelvic osteotomy was delayed when there was little apparent radiological dysplasia a year from reduction; but it was learned that such a delay often led to a mild degree of coxa magna, which eventually lowered the outcome of treatment to Grade 2 rather than Grade 1. So pelvic osteotomy became a routine procedure in all patients. Perhaps it might be felt that this was over-treating the series, but in retrospect we were never disappointed with the results of pelvic osteotomy. Yet when it was delayed, for a good reason, a perfect result was rarely attained.

The overall figures revealed that of the 100 hips assessed, 94% had satisfactory results, including 75 Grade 1 and 19 Grade 2 results. There were six failures, three being unilateral cases of CDH and the other three in bilateral cases. The outcome of these six failures was Grade 4, although they were all salvaged later by a repeat pelvic osteotomy which reduced them to Grade 2, but they were still counted as failures of primary treatment. Sometimes the repeat pelvic osteotomy was delayed until the patient was 10 years old, because of late subluxation developing at that time.

Factors Influencing Outcome. When assessing the results of conservative treatment, in 1960, it was found that in unilateral cases with evidence of dysplasia in the contra-lateral hip joint, the results were unsatisfactory. This was thought to be due to a genetic acetabular dysplasia affecting both hips equally and lowering the potential for recovery on the dislocated side. The same could be said for the

majority of bilateral cases. The influence of this factor was plotted against the degree of acetabular slope in the non-dislocated hip in unilateral cases. Normal values were obtained in patients without dislocations and first and second standard deviations were estimated at various age levels between 5 and 40 months, as seen in Fig. 4.5 on p. 46. The scatter diagrams were found to be different for girls and boys. In both sexes the results of conservative management in unilateral dislocations of the hip were closely related to the degree of dysplasia in the contralateral hip, as seen in Fig. 6.42. When the latter measured more than two standard deviations, the majority of results were failures; but if a contralateral hip was normal and its measurements were below the mean, the outcome of conservative treatment was good or excellent.

Since that review another genetic factor, familial joint laxity, has been discovered in a third of girls and three quarters of boys with CDH, as compared to a 7% prevalence in normal children (Carter and Wilkinson 1964b).

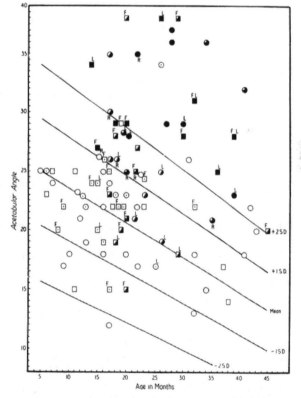

Fig. 6.42. The results of conservative treatment, unilateral CDH, girls, related to the acetabular angle of the non-dislocated hip. Successful:— □ ○ =Grade 1; ▣ ◉ =Grade 2. Intermediate:— ▨ ◑ =Grade 3. Failed:— ▧ ◖ =Grade 4; ■ ● =Grade 5. The greater the angle (above +1 SD and +2 SD), the worse the result. (Carter and Wilkinson 1964b, with permission)

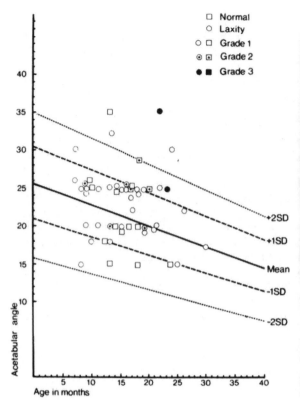

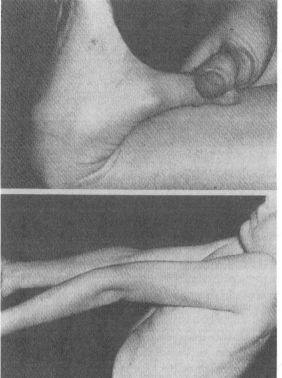

Fig. 6.43. Results of surgical management, unilateral CDH, girls, related to the acetabular angle and familial joint laxity. The poorer results were in those girls with a combination of joint laxity and acetabular dysplasia, both failures being familial cases of CDH.

Fig. 6.44a,b. Signs of familial joint laxity in older children. **a** The thumb test. **b** Hyperextension of the elbows. (Carter and Wilkinson 1964a, with permission)

In the present series the influence of familial joint laxity, in our infant patients, is coupled with the effects of acetabular dysplasia. The combination of these two genetic factors appears to lower the results, even in patients in whom concentric reduction of the hip was attained at an early stage in their management, see Fig. 6.43. The two failed unilateral cases had contralateral hips that were one or two standard deviations above the normal, indicating a marked and severe degree of dysplasia, respectively, combined with a marked degree of familial joint laxity. There were five patients who had a moderate degree of dysplasia in the opposite hip, combined with familial joint laxity, and they ended with Grade 2 results. In only two patients with normal opposite hips combined with familial joint laxity were the results below normal. In other words familial joint laxity, in isolation, did not appear to have a bad influence on the outcome of treatment (see Fig. 6.44).

Thus a combination of severe genetic acetabular dysplasia and familial joint laxity has a bad prognosis, and this coincidence is frequently found in

patients who have an intimate family history of CDH. They have proved to be the most difficult patients to treat in our present series. In such cases the results of early surgical management approach those seen following conservative treatment, but fortunately most of these failures have been salvaged by repeating their pelvic osteotomies at a later stage, as seen in Fig. 6.41.

When there is total paralysis of the pelvifemoral muscle groups, as in poliomyelitis and total paraplegia associated with a meningomyelocele lesion, there is little risk of subluxation or dislocation of the hip joints. Yet cases of partial paralysis, with muscle imbalance, are likely to be complicated by paralytic subluxation and dislocation. It is well known that the combination of paralysed gluteal muscles associated with active flexors and adductor muscles tends to develop paralytic dislocations between the ages of 2 and 6 years, but rarely subsequently. Not only are reduction and the maintenance of stability of the hips difficult, but there is also a high rate of recurrent dislocation if the muscle imbalance is not corrected. In CDH there is a much milder form of muscle imbalance, which may not become apparent until the infants are 2 years old, unless one is aware of such stigmata. These are mild forms of spinal dysraphism and at birth the baby may have a patch of hair or pigmentation, or a lipoma or a post-anal pit in the lumbo-sacral region, as seen in Fig. 4.4 on p. 45. When the patient comes for further assessment, at the age of 2 years, it may be noted that there is wasting of the buttock or the calf muscles. This may be associated with a cavus deformity or inequality of foot size, as seen in Fig. 6.45 (Fairbank 1936). Later the parents may complain of persistent incontinence in the children, and this is sometimes associated with chronic constipation and faecal soiling. There is also a tendency for the children to develop spontaneous fractures of their femurs following a simple injury, especially after the removal of a plaster cast. These supra-condylar fractures are very similar to those sustained in meningomyelocele children, both having a poor prognosis with regard to redisplacement of the hip joint. We are only just becoming aware of such signs in our infant patients who do not respond to our surgical programme. At first the symptoms and signs were thought to be due to prolonged splinting inflicted upon these patients, especially the nocturnal enuresis and constipation. Wasting of the buttock was thought to be the outcome of a poor response to surgery, but retrospectively it becomes apparent that these children were resistant to routine management from the very

beginning. The diagnosis can sometimes be confirmed by straight X-rays of the thoracolumbar region, measuring the interpedicle distance of the vertebrae. Micturating cystograms may reveal the presence of a ureteric reflux, and any suspicion can be confirmed by air myelography.

Such cases are often included in the group of pathological dislocations with arthrogryphosis, mild forms of muscular dystrophy, and rarely patients with familial neuromuscular atrophy. Sometimes the family histories alert the surgeon to an early diagnosis, allowing him to warn the parents of possible complications and err on the side of conservative treatment by delaying surgery for as long as possible.

Summary

1) This personal surgical experience confirms Somerville's findings that 95% of cases of CDH persisting into the second year of life do so because of an incarcerated limbus. Therefore, every infant CDH must be presumed to have such a soft tissue impediment to concentric reduction, before proved otherwise.

2) Eccentric reduction due to soft tissue impediment must now be considered the commonest cause of iatrogenic avascular necrosis in infant patients.

3) Abduction splints should not be applied until concentric reduction has been obtained.

4) Delaying the surgical correction of bony incongruity for 6–12 months from surgical reduction lowers the morbidity complicating management.

5) At the time of surgical reorientation of the bony components, to gain congruity in extension and medial rotation, decompression of the hip joint should also be attained.

6) Uncontrollable factors influencing the outcome of surgical treatment include genetic acetabular dysplasia, familial joint laxity and the muscle imbalance of spinal dysraphism. These factors "will continue to challenge the ingenuity of orthopaedic surgeons for generations to come" (Ortolani 1978).

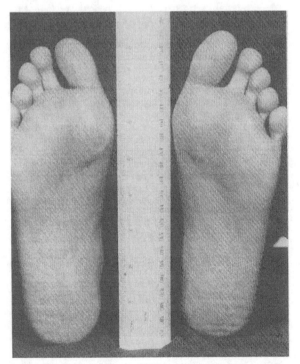

Fig. 6.45. Foot inequality in CDH. As in this patient, the smaller foot is not always on the side of dislocation (left CDH).

References

Badgeley CE (1949) Etiology of congenital dislocation of the hip. J Bone Joint Surg 31A:341

Barnes JM (1980) Premature epiphyseal closure in Perthe's disease. J Bone Joint Surg 62B(4):432

Batchelor JS (1959) Congenital dislocation of the hip. Proc R Soc Med 52:910

Bigelow HJ (1844) quoted by Vernon L Hart (1948) Congenital dysplasia of the hip joint. Charles E. Thomas, Illinois

Borack, Goldhamer (1925) quoted by Severin (1941) Contribution to the knowledge of congenital dislocation of the hip joint. Acta Chir Scand 84, Supplement 63

Bryant T (1880) On the value of parallelism in the lower extremities in the treatment of hip disease and hip injuries with the best means of maintaining it. Lancet 1:159

Bucholz R, Ogden J (1978) Patterns of ischaemic necrosis of the proximal femur in non-operatively treated congenital hip disease. Frank E. Stinchfield Award Paper, Chap. 2. Proceedings of the 6th Open Scientific Meeting of the Hip Society, St. Louis

Caffey J, Ames R, Silverman NA, Ryder CT, Hough G (1956) Contradiction of the congenital dysplasia—pre-dislocation hypothesis of congenital dislocation of the hip through a study of the normal variation in acetabular angles at successive periods in infancy. Pediatrica 17:632

Carter CO, Wilkinson JA (1964a) Genetic and environmental factors in the aetiology of congenital dislocation of the hip. Clin Orthop 33:119

Carter CO, Wilkinson JA (1964b) Persistent joint laxity and congenital displacement of the hip. J Bone Joint Surg 46B

Catford JA, Bennet GC, Wilkinson JA (1982) Congenital dislocation: an increasing and still uncontrolled disability? Br Med J 285:1527

Chuinard EG (1978) Lateral roentgenography in the diagnosis and treatment of dysplasia/dislocation of the hip. Orthopaedics 1:130

Clark KC (1980) Positioning in radiography. Heinemann, London

Coonse GK (1931) A simple modification of Perthe's splint for the early treatment of congenital dislocation of the hip. J Bone Joint Surg XIII:602

David TJ, Parris M, Poynor MU, Simm SA, Hawnaur JM, Rigg EA (1983) Reasons for late detection of hip dislocation in childhood. Lancet 2:147

Davis GG (1903) quoted by Nathanial Allison (1928) Open operations for congenital dislocation of the hip. Robert Jones Birthday Volume, Oxford University Press, Oxford.

Elmslie RC (1913) quoted by Sir Thomas Fairbank (1928) in the Robert Jones Birthday Volume, Oxford University Press, Oxford

Faber A (1937) Erbbiologische Untersuchungen über die Anlage zur "angeborenen" Huftverrenkung. Z Orthop LXVI:140

Fairbank HAT (1928) Infantile or cervical coxa vara. Robert Jones Birthday Volume, Oxford University Press, Oxford

Fairbank HAT (1928) The diagnosis of a limp with special reference to the hip joint. Lancet 1:19–23

Fairbank HAT (1934) Congenital dislocation of the hip. Cambridge University Medical Society Magazine 11:133

Fairbank HAT (1936) Congenital dislocation of the hip. Medical Press and Circular 192:7–10

Fergusson AB (1973) Primary open reduction of congenital dislocation of the hip using a median adductor approach. J Bone Joint Surg 55A:671–689

Gocht (1908) quoted by Severin (1941) Contribution to the knowledge of congenital dislocation of the hip joint. Acta Chir Scand 84, Supplement 63

Haggarty RJ, Moroney MW, Naddis AS (1956) Essential

hypertension in infancy and childhood. Am J Dis Child 92:535–549

Hall G (1981) Some observations of Perthe's disease. J Bone Joint Surg 63B:631

Hart V (1948) Congenital dysplasia of the hip joint and sequelae. Charles E Thomas, Illinois

Hey Groves E (1928) The treatment of congenital dislocation of the hip. Robert Jones Birthday Volume, Oxford University Press, Oxford

Hilgenreiner H (1925) On the early diagnaosis and treatment of congenital dislocation of the hip. Med Klin 21:1385

Howorth MB (1947) Congenital dislocation of the hip. Ann Surg 125:216–236

Judet J (1958) L'Avenir des luxations congénitales de la hanche réduites. Rev Chir Orthop 44:152

Le Damany P (1908) Die angeborene Huftgelenksverrenkung. Z Orthop Chir 21:129

Lehman WB (1980) Early soft-tissue release in congenital dislocation of the hip. Isr J Med Sci 16(4):267

Le Veuf J (1947) Primary congenital subluxation of the hip. J Bone Joint Surg 29:149–162

Le Veuf J (1948) Results of open reduction of true congenital luxation of the hip. J Bone Joint Surg 30A:875

Lloyd-Roberts GC (1971) Orthopaedics in infancy and childhood, 1st edn, chap 13, p 213. Butterworths, London

Lloyd-Roberts GC, Swann M (1966) Pitfalls in the management of congenital dislocation of the hip. J Bone Joint Surg 48B(4):666

Lorenz A (1895) quoted by Nathanial Allison (1928) The open operations for congenital dislocation of the hip. Robert Jones Birthday Volume, Oxford University Press, Oxford

Lorenz A (1920) Die sogenannte angeborene Huftverennkung. Enke, Stuttgart

Ludloff K (1913) The open reduction of the congenital hip dislocation by an anterior incision. Am J Surg 10:438–454

MacKenzie IG (1972) Congenital dislocation of the hip: the development of a regional service. J Bone Joint Surg 54B:18

MacKenzie IG, Seddon H, Trevor D (1960) Congenital dislocation of the hip. J Bone Joint Surg 62B:689

Massie WK (1951) Vascular epiphyseal changes in congenital dislocation of the hip. J Bone Joint Surg 33A:284

Massie WK, Howorth MB (1950) Congenital dislocation of the hip. J Bone Joint Surg 32A:519

Maw H, Dorr WM, Henkel L, Lutsche J (1971) Open reduction of congenital dislocation of the hip by Ludloff's method. J Bone Joint Surg 53A:1281–1288

McEwen D (1978) Residual dysplasia and subluxation in congenital dislocation of the hip. J Bone Joint Surg 60B(3):436

McFarland B (1956) Some observations on congenital dislocation of the hip. In: The Sir Thomas Fairbank Birthday Volume, Oxford University Press, Oxford

Mitchell GP (1972) Problems in the early diagnosis and management of congenital dislocation of the hip. J Bone Joint Surg 54B:4

Mitchell GP (1979) Acquired dislocation of the hip in septic arthritis in infancy. J Bone Joint Surg 61B(4):514

Mitchell GP (1984) In discussion, on a paper entitled: Periosteal division in the management of the short leg in childhood. J Bone Joint Surg 66B(2):276

Monk J (1981) The problems of early diagnosis and prevention of congenital dislocation of the hip. J Maternal Child Health, February:76–85

Nicholson JT, Foster RM, Heath RD (1955) Bryant's traction: a provocative cause of circulatory complications. JAMA 157:415–418

Offierski CM (1981) Traumatic dislocation of the hip in children. J Bone Joint Surg 63B(2):194

Ortolani M (1948) La lussazione congenita dell'anca: Nuovi

criteri diagnostici e profilattico-correttivi. Cappelli, Bologna

Ortolani M (1978) Detecting the dislocated hip. Correspondence in the Lancet, March 4th

Paci A (1887) Nuova contributa alla patologia della lussazione iliaca del femore.Archive ed Atti della Società Italiana de Chir 3:444

Palmen K (1961) Preluxation of the hip joint. Acta Paediatr 50, Supplement 129

Perkins G (1928) Signs by which to diagnose congenital dislocation of the hip. Lancet 1:648–650

Platt H (1953) Congenital dislocation of the hip. J Bone Joint Surg Editorial 35B:339

Poggi A (1888) Contributo alla cura cruenta della lussatione congenital. Arch Orthop 105

Putti V (1929) Early treatment of congenital dislocation of the hip. J Bone Joint Surg 11:798–809

Putti V (1933) Early treatment of congenital dislocation of the hip. J Bone Joint Surg 15:16–21

Putti V (1937) Die Anatomie der angeborenen Huftverrenkung. Enke, Stuttgart

Ridlon J (1906) Spontaneous dislocation at the hip joint. Surg Gynecol Obstet 2:613–617

Roentgen WC (1895) Ueber eine neue Art von Strahlen (vorlaeufige Mitteilung). Sitzungs-Berichte der Physikalisch-medizinischen Gesellschaft zu Würzburg 9:132

Salter RB (1961) Innominate osteotomy in the treatment of congenital dislocation and subluxation of the hip. J Bone Joint Surg 43B:518

Salter RB (1983) Combined open reduction and innominate osteotomy for congenital dislocation of the hip. Strategies Orthop Surg 2(4) May

Salter RB, Kostuick J, Dallas S (1969) Avascular necrosis of the femoral head as a complication of treatment for congenital dislocation of the hip in young children. Can J Surg 12:44

Scaglietti O, Calandriello B (1962) Open reduction of congenital dislocation of the hip. J Bone Joint Surg 44B:257

Schneider M (1962) Femoral torsion: an experimental study. J Bone Joint Surg 44A:1021

Scott JC (1953) Frame reduction in congenital dislocation of the hip. J Bone Joint Surg 35B:372

Severin E (1941) Contribution to the knowledge of congenital dislocation of the hip joint. Acta Chir Scand 84, Supplement 63

Shenton EWH (1911) Disease in bone and its detection by the X-rays. Macmillan, London

Smith T (1874) Acute arthritis of infants. St. Bartholomew's Report 10:189–204

Somerville EW (1953) Development of congenital dislocation of the hip. J Bone Joint Surg 35B:363

Somerville EW, Scott JC (1957) The direct approach to congenital dislocation of the hip. J Bone Joint Surg 39B:623

Soutter R (1914) A new operation for hip contractures in poliomyelitis. Boston Med Surg J 170:380

Steiner RE (1983) Nuclear magnetic resonance: its clinical application. J Bone Joint Surg 65B(5):533–535

Stewart WJ (1934) Further observations on the abduction-traction treatment of congenital dislocation of the hip. J Bone Joint Surg 16:303

Tanner JM, Whitehouse RH, Takaishi M (1966) Standards from birth to maturity for height, weight, height velocity and weight velocity in British children in 1965. Arch Dis Child 41:613–635

Tonnis D (1976) An evaluation of conservative and operative methods in the treatment of congenital hip dislocation. Clin Orthop 119:76

Tonnis D (1982) Congenital hip dislocation—avascular necrosis. Thieme-Stratton, New York

Truetta A (1968) Studies of the development and decay of the human frame. Heinemann, London

Tsuchiya K, Yamanda K (1978) Open reduction of congenital dislocation of the hip in infancy using Ludloff's approach. Int Orthop (SICOT) 1:337

Tucker FR (1949) Arterial supply to the femoral head and its clinical importance. J Bone Joint Surg 31B:82

Vickers RH, Catterall A (1980) A trial of closed reduction: a method of management in congenital dislocation of the hip under the age of 2. J Bone Joint Surg 62B:526

Weiner DS, Cook AJ (1980) Practical considerations in the use of computed tomography in the measurement of femoral anteversion. Isr J Med Sci 16(4):288

Weiner DS, Cook AJ, Hoyt WA, Oravec CE (1978) Computed tomography in the measurement of femoral anteversion. Orthopaedics 1(4):299

Weinstein SL (1980) The medical approach in congenital dislocation of the hip. Isr J Med Sci 16(4):272

Weintroub S, Boyde A, Chrispin RA, Lloyd-Roberts GC (1981) The use of stereophotogrammetry to measure acetabular and femoral anteversion. J Bone Joint Surg 63B(2):209

Wiberg G (1939) Studies on dysplastic acetabula and congenital subluxation of the hip joint. Acta Chir Scand 83, Supplement 58

Wilkinson JA (1972) A post-natal survey for congenital dislocation of the hip. J Bone Joint Surg 54B:40

Wilkinson JA (1980) Results of surgical treatment in congenital dislocation of the hip. Isr J Med Sci 16:281–283

Wilkinson JA (1982) The surgical treatment of congenital dislocation of the hip joint. J Bone Joint Surg 64B(5):636

Wilkinson JA, Carter CO (1960) Congenital dislocation of the hip. J Bone Joint Surg 42B:652

Wilkinson JA, Howell CJ (1973) Management of infants with congenital displacement of the hip. Proc R Soc Med 66(3):9–10

7　Juvenile Hip Displacement
($3\frac{1}{2}$ Years to Skeletal Maturity)

> In the treatment of congenital dislocation of the hip we are confronted by a situation unusual in joint dislocations in general—an intra-capsular dislocation in which there is an inherent incongruity between the femoral head and the acetabulum.
>
> *Sir Harry Platt* (1953)

It is surprising that in our modern society there can be children born with CDH which goes undetected until they are at least 3 years old, yet it was little more than 50 years ago that Perkins (1928) wrote that few of his patients with CDH reached the hospital before this age. Even today, every year, two or three patients in this juvenile group are referred for the first time to our service, because of a painless limp in one hip or a waddling gait due to bilateral instability of their hips.

We find that juvenile patients tend to fall into two groups, the smaller containing those that have never been diagnosed previously, but the larger being made up of those children who have been diagnosed and treated unsuccessfully in the earlier part of their lives.

Missed CDH

Perhaps the majority of these cases involve congenital subluxations, which are usually bilateral. This accounts for the delay in diagnosis, because there is little evidence of leg inequality and hip instability. These are not late displacements resulting from persistent instability of their hips due to familial joint laxity and genetic acetabular dysplasia; rather they have been present from birth and are usually complete displacements, in that there is

a soft tissue impediment to concentric reduction. They were described as "tight dislocations", by Mitchell (1963), in which arthrography reveals not only the residual instability and displacement, but also a mechanical acetabular dysplasia secondary to an inverted limbus and a deformed femoral head, as shown in Fig. 7.1. Sometimes complete luxations are first seen at this age, and again they are usually bilateral. This means that the children affected have little leg inequality and present with a waddling gait. It is not unusual for their parents to have been reassured, by previous medical advisers, that this is normal and will correct spontaneously!

Failed Infantile CDH

Unfortunately our larger group of children presenting with residual instability of their hips from congenital causes, after the age of 3 years, are those that have been diagnosed previously and treated in the first and second years of life. Yet for some inexplicable reason they have not been followed up and eventually present at a later date with a limp. Often their parents are bewildered, because they have been assured at an earlier examination that their child will grow up normally. Their doctors have broken the rule that any such patients should be kept under observation at regular intervals of not

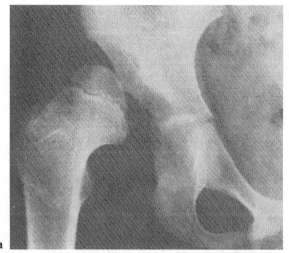
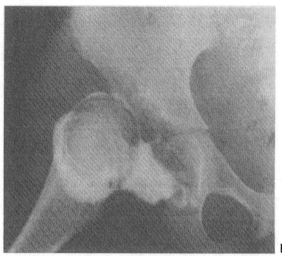

a   t

Fig. 7.1a,b. Juvenile hip subluxation or "tight dislocations". Five-year-old girl. **a** X-ray reveals displacement associated with severe acetabular dysplasia. **b** Arthrogram reveals a large inverted limbus with central pooling. The femoral head appears normal, but the acetabulum is shallow.

more than 12 months, up to the age of 6 years and sometimes even later when there is radiological evidence of persistent dysplasia of the hip joint.

The testing time for juvenile hip stability is between 10 and 12 years. Before the menarche, the blood levels of oestrogens and androgens are slowly raised by pituitary stimulation (Ganong 1973). This coincides with a rapid spurt of skeletal growth (Tanner et al. 1966).

At this period (10–12 years), girls with familial joint laxity can develop the first symptoms and signs of recurrent subluxation of the patellae and shoulders. According to Professor Geoffrey Burwell (personal communication), juvenile scoliosis also begins to develop at this age. All these conditions are the result of rapid growth sometimes combined with familial joint laxity, or are due to the development of hormonal joint laxity in the pre-puberty phase. There are few specialists in this field who have not been confounded by seeing a young woman with residual subluxation or even redislocation of the hips, who had been previously assessed as having a good result from infantile management. The routine review of CDH patients should not be discontinued before skeletal maturity has been attained.

Many of these cases of juvenile CDH have stigmata of iatrogenic deformation, which is not confined to the scarring of the overlying skin. Their hips are sometimes stiff, but they may only complain of fatigue and discomfort following exercise and their inability to keep up with their friends in sporting activities.

Clinical Features

Perkins (1928) pointed out that it is not difficult to miss instability of the hip when the examiner concentrates his attention to the hip level, as he may not observe the limp at all. If, however, he watches the point of the shoulders, the sideways sway of the trunk becomes apparent as the shoulders dip down on the affected side when weight is borne on that leg, as seen in Fig. 7.2. Perkins explained the characteristic gait of CDH as follows:

When the normal individual takes one leg off the ground, say the left, and balances on the other, the weight of the trunk would naturally depress the pelvis on the left side because the supporting leg is not directly under the line of the body-weight. To prevent this, the muscles of the right hip-joint contract strongly and tilt the pelvis down on the right side. This is the normal. If for any reason the abductor muscles lose their powers they cannot tilt the pelvis down on the right side and the body-weight causes the pelvis to tilt down to the left; then the patient, to prevent himelf from falling sideways to the left, throws his trunk over to the right, so that the line of body-weight passes down through the supporting leg. It is the tilt of the trunk towards the affected side when the affected leg is bearing weight that gives the characteristic gait. In a congenital dislocation the abductor muscles, although powerful, are ineffectual, because they lack the fulcrum

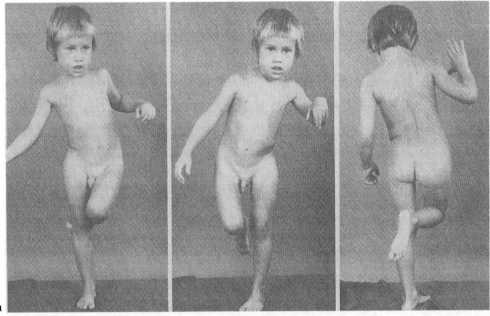

Fig. 7.2a–c. Bilateral juvenile CDH. Five-year-old. X-rays demonstrated in Fig. 7.12. **a** Standing on right leg, his right shoulder drops as he leans to the right to balance his centre of gravity, or he would fall to the left. **b** Standing on left leg, his left shoulder dips. **c** Posteriorly the fold of the right buttock falls, i.e. positive Trendelenburg test first described by Friedrich Trendelenburg (1844–1924).

which normally is supplied by the head of the femur fitting into the acetabulum. (Perkins 1928)

When there is bilateral displacement, the sway is first to one side and then to the other, the gait becoming rolling and more obvious.

Perkins also described the female profile of children with bilateral CDH, produced by the fullness of the lateral outline of the trunk and legs caused by the prominence of the greater trochanters, as compared to the slim-hipped appearance of the normal child, who has a male profile. The umbilicus is another clinical feature, as normally it lies well above the midpoint between the crown and the heel in 2-year-olds; but in bilateral CDH it often lies near or on the midpoint, while in achondroplasia it frequently lies below it. Also the distance between the anterosuperior iliac spine and the tip of the greater trochanter should indicate any displacement when the span is less than normal, whether there be unilateral or bilateral hip involvement (see Fig. 6.3). With the hips and knees flexed, abduction of the hips is severely restricted in these cases owing to secondary contracture of the adductor muscles. There is also a contracture of the hamstrings which may limit straight leg raising when the knees are extended.

Perhaps many of these cases would not be missed if those responsible for the clinical vetting remembered the words of Mitchell (1970), who enlarged on the difficulties of examining a restless infant to exclude bilateral CDH. He advised that an X-ray examination should always be arranged when the mother notices any abnormality of gait, "for this alone will prevent the tragedy of missed bilateral CDH presenting at 4, 6 and 8 years of age".

Radiological Features

The diagnosis should never be in doubt as at this time the femoral head is well ossified, but it may be deformed owing to previous treatment. Shenton's line is often broken due to the upward and lateral drift of the femoral head in residual subluxations, and in complete displacements the femoral head may be seen to lie in a false acetabulum above the anterior inferior iliac spine.

When there is no deformity of the femoral head, it may be difficult to differentiate between a residual displacement and a congenital subluxation. Arth-

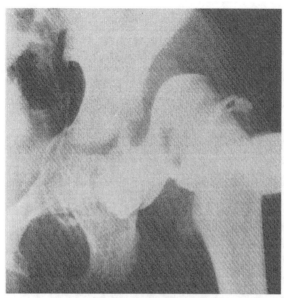

Fig. 7.3. Arthrogram of juvenile CDH, hourglass appearance due to the infolded limbus above and the ileopsoas tendon below the constriction.

1) It is essential to lower the femoral head to the level of the triradiate cartilage, either by pre-operative traction, or by surgical soft tissue release, or both.

2) It is essential to explore and remove all soft tissue impediments in the acetabulum, in order to obtain concentric reduction of the femoral head.

3) It is necessary to produce a bony roof to cover the femoral head and so prevent residual subluxation.

4) Any operative procedure which compresses the hip can only produce deformation of the femoral head and residual incongruity of the articular surfaces, which will lead to an early osteoarthrosis.

Putti (1933) stressed the importance of complete reduction thus:

It is a complete delusion that one can have a result permanently satisfactory in function in a hip incompletely reduced. Every such hip that has not obtained from the first, or not preserved normal anatomical relationship between the femoral epiphysis and the acetabulum, is inevitably destined to become the subject of that precocious articular senility which is usually diagnosed as osteoarthritis. No complete and permanent restoration of function occurs apart from perfect anatomical reduction.

rography will help in these cases, for in congenital subluxation there is usually an incarcerated limbus, as described by Mitchell (1963; see Fig. 7.1).

Arthrography in juvenile CDH often reveals an hourglass appearance due to the infolding of the limbus and capsule from above and the constriction of the tight iliopsoas tendon below, as seen in Fig. 7.3.

Surgical Management

Many of the principles as well as the pitfalls of surgical procedures employed in these patients were discovered and written up in detail by the doyens of orthopaedic surgery at the beginning of this century. Hey Groves (1928) described almost every surgical procedure that is used today, including open surgical reduction, acetabuloplasty, femoral shortening and capsulorrhaphy. Indeed some of the experts in these techniques are still to be found in the middle European countries, where late presentation of CDH is more common; only recently papers have emerged from Yugoslavia, Greece, Italy, and also California, U.S.A.

The principles that are to be observed in such surgery are as follows:

Pre-operative Traction

Although some authorities believe that skeletal traction is likely to be a cause of avascular necrosis in this age group (Westin et al. 1980), most people believe that a period of pre-operative traction does no harm in such cases. Below the age of 4 years it is still possible to apply this vertically, as in the infantile patients described in Chap. 6. The only fear in older children is that of ischaemic damage to their feet, but it is only likely to develop when the infant's legs reach a length of 42 cm (after the age of 4 years according to Tanner 1946 and 1973). In older children, one has to accept a horizontal balanced traction which is applied on a pulley system attached to a bar fitted to the foot of the bed, the latter being elevated 20 cm above the horizontal. This is far less effective, as the iliopsoas contracture has to be overcome, but it is wise to continue such traction methods for a period up to 6 weeks and not to forcibly abduct the legs beyond 50°.

At the end of the traction period, the child is examined under a general anaesthetic. In some of the younger patients, especially those with familial joint laxity, the hip may be found to have become reducible. In this group the femoral head can be felt to jump in and out of the acetabulum, but reduction is usually unstable due to the eccentricity of the femoral head in the acetabulum. David Trevor (1957) emphasised that although excision of part or all of the limbus allows eccentric reduction to be converted easily and safely to a concentric one, "a truly irreducible dislocation, in which the head will not descend to the level of the acetabulum or enter it, can never be reduced by the simple means of removing the inverted limbus". Yet in children under the age of $3\frac{1}{2}$, when the hip is reducible, it is possible to perform a posterior arthrotomy in order to remove the limbus and plicate the excess capsule. The child is then splinted in a Lorenz plaster and later a Denis Browne harness, to continue with the same management that is carried out on infant cases under the age of 3 years. In the majority of juvenile patients, however, the hip will be found to be irreducible at the end of traction and it is then necessary to resort to open reduction at this stage.

Open Reduction

When the hip is irreducible, it is necessary to perform an extensive open reduction through an anterosuperior approach in preference to the restricted posterior arthrotomy. The Salter approach (1961) has been employed in this series, using an incision extending from the mid-inguinal point horizontally to a point distal to the middle of the iliac crest. The incision is deepened through the fatty layer of the subcutaneous tissue and then between its fascial layer and the deep fascia itself, dissecting upward to expose the iliac crest. The anterior aspect of the hip joint is approached between the tensor fascia lata and the sartorius, lateral to the lateral cutaneous nerve, which is preserved and retracted medially. The incision is deepened to expose the antero-inferior iliac spine, identifying the origin of the straight head of the rectus femoris. The iliac apophysis is then split longitudinally, down to the bone, along the iliac crest from the anterosuperior iliac spine to the tubercle of the crest and posteriorly as far as possible. The two halves of the apophysis are then separated with the attached periosteum, which is stripped from both the outer and inner surfaces of the ilium as far back as the greater sciatic notch. On the outer aspect, the periosteum is stripped down to the attachment of the capsular ligament of the hip joint, and at this level the periosteum is incised to reveal the anterosuperior aspect of the capsule. It is not unusual to find the superior capsule adherent to the lateral aspect of the ilium (Trevor 1960), and this adherence should be stripped to the original level of its attachment just superior to the bony rim of the acetabulum. The capsule is then incised parallel to, but 1 cm lateral to its acetabular attachment, opening the false capsular acetabulum to expose the contained femoral head. An elongated ligamentum teres can usually be seen stretching from the fovea of the head to the site of the original bony acetabulum. The anatomical variations discovered in these cases have been recorded previously by many authorities, but none of the descriptions are more detailed than those of David Trevor (1960) and Scaglietti and Calandrillo (1962), as they were master surgeons in this field.

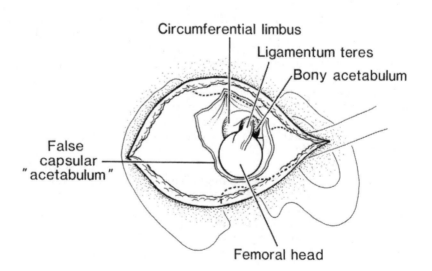

Fig. 7.4. Intracapsular appearance in juvenile CDH. Note the circumferential limbus covering the acetabulum, its central hiatus allowing the elongated ligamentum teres to extend from the head of the femur to the floor of the bony acetabulum.

Circumferential limbus

Ligamentum teres

Bony acetabulum

False capsular "acetabulum"

Femoral head

Capsular Features. In the capsule covering the displaced femoral head and forming a false acetabulum, the fibres run from the posterior rim of the acetabulum over the femoral head to be inserted into the anterior aspect of the intertrochanteric line, as described in Chap. 3. The capsular hood is often adherent to the external surface of the ilium and has to be stripped down to reveal its original attachment to the acetabular rim. When the joint is opened, the capsule forming the false acetabulum is found to extend downwards to become continuous with the limbus which infolds and restricts the approach to the bony acetabulum (see Fig. 7.4). Sometimes it almost covers completely the acetabular opening, except for a small hiatus through which the ligamentum teres extends and this anatomical feature can be used to locate the bony acetabulum. A blunt hook inserted through the central hiatus can be used to palpate the outer edge of the articular surface indicating the base of the rolled limbus. A circumferential incision made along the articular edge is used to excise the limbus and expose the true bony acetabulum underneath. The ligamentum teres is usually present in luxations, but sometimes absent in subluxations (Le Veuf 1948). When present, it is usually stretched and attenuated and sometimes bifid.

Bony Features. The normal spherical appearance of the femoral head is usually replaced by an ovoid or hemispherical shape that has been described as a "lozenge" or "olive". Its summit may be difficult to identify, but can be recognised by the fovea from which emerges the ligamentum teres. Once located, it helps in the measurement of any degree of anteversion or retroversion that may be present. At this age the femoral neck is usually anteverted, but even with this extensive exposure it is often difficult to measure the degree of femoral torsion, and occasionally one is surprised to find a marked degree of retroversion.

Once the limbus has been excised and the acetabulum exposed, it is usual to find the latter to be normal in shape and depth, big enough to contain what appears to be an enlarged femoral head. It is necessary to recognise the inferior extension of the limbus which can restrict the opening of the acetabulum and should be excised. Some people refer to this part of the limbus as the "transverse ligament of the acetabulum".

Location of the femoral head is not difficult once any soft tissue impediment has been removed and it must be rare to find the femoral head to be too large for the acetabulum. The ligamentum teres never appears to cause any obstruction to this reduction and it should not be removed, as it contracts down post-operatively and creates a natural attachment for the femoral head, preventing any lateral drift.

In two patients, the acetabulum was found to be virtually absent and could only be recognised as a small shallow impression at the level of the triradiate cartilage, and in each case the femoral head appeared of normal size.

Extra-articular Contractures. The persistence of hip displacement during the first 3 years of life or more leads to contractures developing in the deep fascia and the pelvifemoral muscle groups. This affects mainly the tensor fascia lata and gluteus medius, and also the iliopsoas and adductor muscles. In older children the hamstring muscles are also involved. Such contractures are strong enough to prevent reduction of the femoral head. Even in those cases where reduction has been attained, they may cause compression of the articular surfaces leading to post-operative stiffness and late epiphyseal fragmentation and compression.

The Salter approach involves the stripping of the outer and inner surfaces of the ilium, releasing any contractures of the abductors and iliopsoas. This facilitates the reduction of the femoral head.

Femoral Osteotomy

The success of femoral shortening in the reduction of a dislocated femoral head in this age group has already been mentioned. It is a well-tried procedure and was originally described by Hey Groves (1928) who performed it through a Lorenz bifurcation subtrochanteric osteotomy, which was an oblique osteotomy of the femoral shaft in the subtrochanteric region displacing the distal fragment medially and allowing the two fragments to override:

The osteotomy is done through a small lateral incision on the thigh, just on the level with the antero-inferior iliac spine. The bone is cut through in an oblique direction downwards and backwards so as to give as broad overlapping surfaces of raw bone as possible. After dividing the bone, the leg is forcibly abducted and then the shaft of the femur is thrust towards the acetabulum, this position being maintained by a plaster spica. When union of the bone has been effected the upper end of the femur represents a 'Y' shaped or bifurcated end which affords a sort of crutch upon which the pelvis rests.

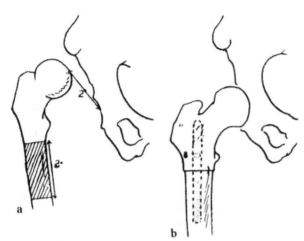

Fig. 7.5a,b. Hey-Groves' original diagram of femoral shortening to reduce a juvenile CDH. (Hey Groves 1928, with permission)

Later Hey Groves developed another technique of femoral shortening, removing 2 or 3 in. of the femoral shaft in order to bring the head of the femur down to the level of the acetabulum, as shown in Fig. 7.5.

Femoral shortening for the surgical reduction of CDH in patients above the age of 3½–4 years has retained its popularity in many countries. Dega et al. (1959) described a technique in children between 3 and 5 years, where subtrochanteric osteotomy was employed to shorten the femur 1–3 cm and derotate any excess anteversion, in order to bring the femoral head down to the site of the primary acetabulum. They used it in association with a Hey Groves capsuloplasty, later popularised by Colonna (1932) in older children. Westin et al. (1980) found that their technique of femoral shortening was far preferable to skeletal traction in reduction of CDH in older children. They used their technique of a sliding osteotomy in cases up to the age of puberty. This was very similar to the Lorenz bifurcation osteotomy, but they used it in association with open reduction of the hip and fixation, by inserting a Steinman's pin through the greater trochanter and into the pelvis above the acetabulum. They allowed the osteotomy to adjust itself in a plaster spica.

The technique of open reduction, femoral shortening and at the same time correcting any increase of femoral anteversion has been used successfully, either combined with pelvic osteotomy at the same time or followed by the same procedure 4–6 weeks later, in both congenital subluxations and dislocations, as seen in Figs. 7.12 and 7.13.

Such surgery is courageous and one is dependent upon normal muscle development and balance in order to stabilise the femoral head.

Acetabular Reconstruction

In this group, the persistent displacement of the femoral head out of the acetabulum produces a severe secondary mechanical dysplasia. There is usually a severe degree of shelving of the acetabular roof in congenital subluxations, whereas the femoral head may lie higher in a false acetabulum in persistent luxations. In both cases there may be thickening of the bony floor of the acetabulum which increases the degree of shallowness of the socket. These changes produce a varying degree of instability of the femoral head.

The history of paediatric orthopaedics is littered with the various techniques used in order to stabilise such hip joints. As already mentioned, Hey Groves (1928) developed the technique of gouging the floor of the acetabulum away, to produce a sufficient depth to contain the femoral head, then wrapping the latter in the whole of the capsule, which is detached from the rim of the socket and used to anchor the femoral head in its new bed. This form of capsular arthroplasty was later developed by Colonna (1953), David Trevor (1960) and Sir Harry Platt (reported by Glass and Dunningham 1980). Glass and Dunningham quoted Lloyd-Roberts (1978), who believed the Hey Groves/Colonna capsular arthroplasty to have been superseded by other techniques, but Pipino (1980) used the same operation associated with a Chiari medial displacement osteotomy of the femur in order to stabilise the congenital displacements of 6–26 year olds in Italy and he gained some degree of success.

Acetabuloplasty. The method of turning down a flap of bone from the outer surface of the ilium in order to stabilise a residual subluxation of the hip was also developed by Hey Groves (1928) and he laid down the three principles for success:

1) The bone flap must be massive, consisting of the whole outer table of the ilium, otherwise it would be absorbed.

2) It must be secured in place, so that it shall remain jutting out over the socket.

3) The bone flap must be turned down to the level of the natural rim of the acetabulum, otherwise it will allow the head of the femur to ride up outside its proper socket.

His techniques were developed at the Lord Mayor Treloar Orthopaedic Hospital by his colleage, Sir Thomas Fairbank, whose skill and influence led Bryan McFarland (1956) to refer to the operative procedure as the "Fairbank shelf operation"; I am indebted to Dr Ronald Murray for the original X-rays of one of his patients, shown in Fig. 7.6. This form of acetabuloplasty has persisted and it is still an excellent way of maintaining concentric reduction of the femoral head by stimulating the development of the acetabular roof.

David Trevor (1960) pointed out that spontaneous recovery of acetabular dysplasia did not always follow concentric reduction of the femoral head and that infrequently acetabuloplasty was required in the young when open replacement was unstable due to a shallow roof, but in the older child with a more advanced degree of mechanical dysplasia there is an appreciable lag in the ossification of the cartilage of the acetabular roof. He found that replacement of the femoral head after 3 years of age, under such circumstances, hardly ever allows a natural speed-up of roof ossification, so that the potential danger of redislocation is very real. He performed acetabuloplasty as an extra-articular procedure, whereby the roof is turned over a concentrically placed femoral head in a swing fashion, the fulcrum being at a point on the inner pelvic wall just above the acetabulum: "It should extend from just above the anterior margin right .back to the posterior margin towards the sciatic notch and should be deep enough to penetrate the pelvic wall in order to produce a full swing downward".

Pemberton (1965) described a similar acetabuloplasty to correct the anterior subluxation produced by a defect in the anterior border of the acetabulum. He also felt that this restricted the acetabular space, which was always larger in these older children as compared to the smaller femoral head. His osteotomy extended from above the acetabulum backwards into the posterior limb of the triradiate cartilage, which had sufficient plasticity to permit downward and lateral displacement.

Our experience of acetabuloplasty is that it produces stiff hips and sometimes coxa plana, due to the fact that there is no element of decompression in this operative procedure. There is also no element of reorientation of the acetabulum, from its retroverted position to the normal anteverted site, and this means that sometimes late residual subluxation takes place (see Fig. 7.7). Thus pelvic osteotomy has superseded acetabuloplasty, as it is a safer procedure and it not only decompresses, but reorientates the acetabulum to its normal anatomical position.

Chiari Osteotomy. In severe residual subluxation the femoral head lies in a false acetabulum above the anterior inferior iliac spine. If it is not possible to reduce the femoral head by abduction of the hip, then it is almost certain that a pelvic osteotomy will displace the femoral head more laterally and increase the degree of instability. Pelvic osteotomy with lateral and anterior displacement can only be successful when the femoral head is reduced into the primary acetabulum.

A number of techniques have been developed to accommodate those cases with persistent eccentric reduction, and Chiari osteotomy is one such procedure. The technique was developed in 1950 with

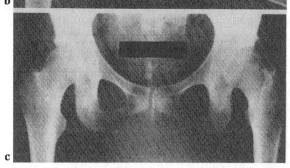

Fig. 7.6a–c. The "Fairbank shelf operation" or acetabuloplasty. **a** Juvenile left CDH treated by Sir Thomas in 1943. **b** Surgical reduction and stabilisation by acetabuloplasty, 1945. **c** 15-year follow-up X-rays, 1960 (from the Radiological Archives, Lord Mayor Treloar Hospital, Alton, by kind permission of Dr Ronald Murray).

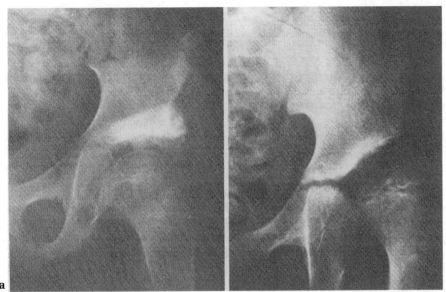

Fig. 7.7a,b. Long-term follow-up after acetabuloplasty. **a** Acetabuloplasty for residual subluxation in 3-year-old girl, 1960. **b** Same patient in 1968, complaining of discomfort and fatigue in left hip.

the intention of improving on the results of the old "shelf" operations. Through an iliofemoral approach an osteotomy is performed in an oblique manner in order to promote medial displacement of the acetabulum, the upper pelvic fragment providing a new roof to the socket. Chiari (1955) described it as an extra-articular procedure with the idea that the superior capsule lies between the femoral head and the buttress of bone, as seen in Fig. 7.8. Although this is an excellent technique for stabilising a residual subluxation of the joint, and it is usually followed by a remarkable degree of remodelling

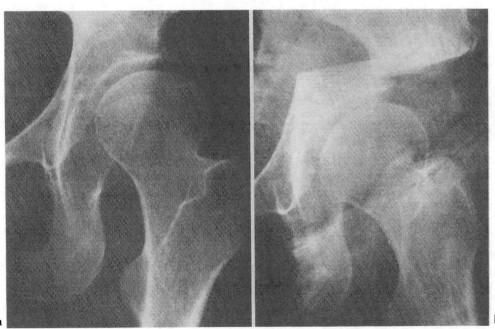

Fig. 7.8a,b. Chiari osteotomy reserved for patients in whom concentric reduction of the femoral head cannot be easily obtained, because it lies in a false acetabulum. **a** Subluxated femoral head in adult. **b** Post-operative X-ray—Chiari osteotomy.

of the acetabulum and pelvis to provide an adequate socket for the femoral head, there are two residual problems with the procedure:

1) The child is left with a permanent limp and this is probably biomechanical, due to a shortening of the leverage of the abductors on the greater trochanter, caused by the medial displacement of the weight-bearing area of the hip joint toward the midline.

2) If the procedure is performed in children between the ages of 4 and 8 years, the triradiate cartilage continues to grow, causing an upward migration of the acetabular roof, which eventually leads to a persistent subluxation of the femoral head, as shown in Fig. 7.9.

Thus a Chiari osteotomy is a very effective way of stabilising the hip joint in a mature patient. It produces a relief of pain with the retention of an excellent range of movement. The result is only scarred by a persistent dipping gait, which cannot be corrected by transplanting the greater trochanter distally. The procedure should never be used in the younger age group for the reasons given. Similarly we have found that in some patients who have had a pelvic osteotomy with lateral and forward displacement of the distal fragment, extrusion of the fixation pins can produce a collapse of the graft and residual

medial displacement of the lower segment mimicking a Chiari-type procedure. If such a result is accepted, further subluxation of the hip will occur as the triradiate cartilage contributes to the growth of the pelvis, and the long-term result will be poor. We have learned to our cost that any collapse of the graft should be corrected immediately, but the complication has not occurred since we have adopted the use of two internal fixation pins rather than a single one.

Triple Osteotomy of the Innominate Bone. This was a technique developed by Steele (1973) in 7–17-year-old patients in whom it was not possible to reduce the hip concentrically and stabilise it with any form of single pelvic osteotomy.

The procedure involved a triple osteotomy including the ischeal tuberosity, the superior pubic ramus, and the ilium just above the acetabulum. A modified technique of triple pelvic osteotomy was described by Tonnis et al. (1981), in which they performed a spherical osteotomy around the acetabulum in order to rotate it freely over the head of the femur. It is necessary to transfix the iliac osteotomy and sometimes to insert a triangle graft to keep it in its new position.

All these techniques stabilise the head in an eccentric position, as they do not attempt to lower the femoral head to the site of the original

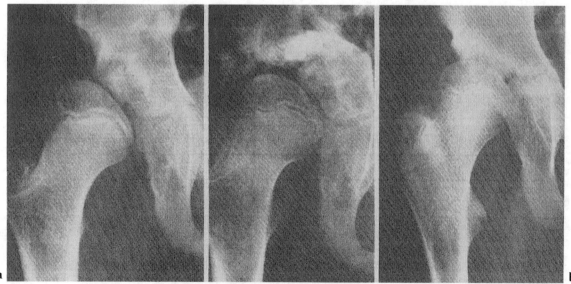

a   b, c

Fig. 7.9a–c. Juvenile subluxation—Chiari osteotomy. **a** Six-year-old girl with congenital subluxation. **b** Same patient 1 year after Chiari osteotomy. **c** Same patient 4 years after Chiari osteotomy with some discomfort and severe limp due to positive Trendelenburg test. Note the residual subluxation of the hip.

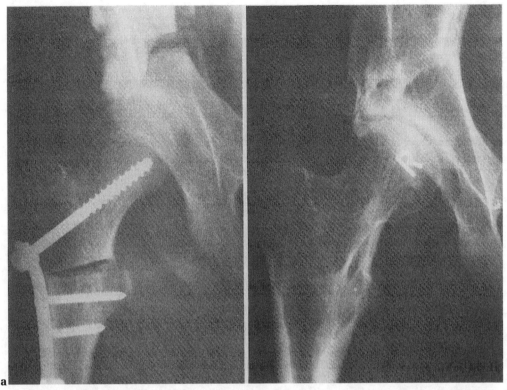

a   b

Fig. 7.10a,b. Residual subluxation in juvenile treated by femoral shortening and pelvic osteotomy. **a** Same 10-year-old patient as in Fig. 7.9c. Residual subluxation corrected by 2 cm of femoral shortening followed by pelvic osteotomy. **b** Four years later—no pain or limp and full range of hip movements.

acetabulum, although Steele did apply pre-operative skeletal traction and extensive soft tissue release with this intention. The failure rate of such surgery is usually between 20% and 30% and there are many complications.

It is felt that the results of these multiple osteotomies of the pelvis are not comparable to the combined femoral shortening and pelvic osteotomy, for when this procedure is performed efficiently it produces a concentric reduction of the hip in its normal situation, even in the most resistant cases, as shown in Fig. 7.10.

Southampton Management of Late CDH

In all patients over 3 years of age, primary closed reduction is likely to be more traumatic than open reduction and the same is probably true for children below 2 years of age. Forcible manipulation can easily cause epiphysitis even after a period on traction on a frame and metaphyseal changes can occur as well. (A. L. Eyre-Brook 1966)

It is essential to stabilise the femoral head at the site of the original acetabulum, in order to stimulate normal growth in the triradiate cartilage and ensure normal development of the acetabulum subsequently. The sensitivity of the triradiate growth plate to distorting forces was well demonstrated experimentally in Chap. 2. This fact might well account for the success of Salter's pelvic osteotomy and the failure of the Chiari osteotomy in the growing child. The former procedure rotates the triradiate growth plate to its normal frontal and horizontal position, whereas the Chiari osteotomy displaces it vertically (as seen in Fig. 7.9) and this is the cause of late subluxation.

Combined Pelvic and Femoral Osteotomies. The hip is first approached through a Salter incision, mobilising the origins of the abductors and flexors on the outer and inner side of the pelvis, respectively, with a view to finally sliding their sites of origin distally. This preserves their tendons of insertion with the pedicle blood supply to the proximal third of the femur through the lesser and greater trochanters. An extensive arthrotomy will provide the access to deal with any soft tissue impediment to concentric reduction, and also to strip any high attachment of the capsule to the outer aspect of the ilium, so preventing any residual subluxation of the femoral head.

At this stage, a preconceived degree of femoral shortening (as measured from the distance between the calcar of the displaced femur to the lower border of the superior pubic ramus) must be performed in order to re-establish Shenton's line. It is better to fix the proximal and distal femoral fragments, using a Coventry screw and plate fixation technique, as this will also allow any correction of excessive femoral torsion and coxa valga. Then the femoral head can be placed in the primary acetabulum easily and without any compression. Finally a pelvic osteotomy must be performed, to rotate the shallow

acetabulum laterally and anteriorly in order to stabilise the femoral head. The two halves of the iliac apophysis are then approximated without tension, the upper third of the iliac crest being excised previously (see Chap. 6).

Such principles must be obeyed in the treatment of juvenile congenital subluxation and luxation. In the former the degree of femoral shortening is not excessive, but it is still important, for if the femoral head is not lowered to the site of the primary acetabulum, the subsequent pelvic osteotomy will only displace the femoral head laterally, aggravating the degree of instability. This technique is shown

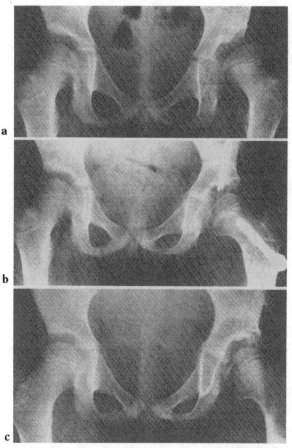

Fig. 7.11a–c. Juvenile hip subluxation in 5-year-old girl. **a** Pre-operative X-ray, the horizontal lines indicating the required length of femoral shortening. **b** Post-operative X-ray following open reduction and excision of the limbus, femoral osteotomy and 2 cm of shortening, and pelvic osteotomy. **c** 3 years later, excellent result.

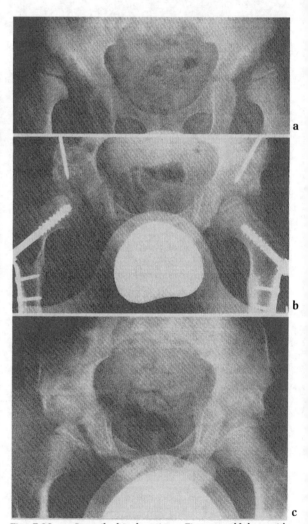

Fig. 7.12a–c. Juvenile hip luxations. Five-year-old boy with bilateral CDH not previously diagnosed or treated. **a** X-ray when first seen. Clinical photographs in Fig. 7.2. **b** A year later, following two-stage open reduction, femoral shortening (2 cm) and pelvic osteotomies. **c** Two years later, walking without a limp and no stiffness.

in Fig. 7.11. In residual luxations, the same principles must be heeded even more urgently, or redislocation will occur and the child will not benefit. The results of such surgery can be seen in Fig. 7.12. In cases of residual subluxation, due to failure of earlier treatment, it is more difficult to correct iatrogenic deformity of the femoral head and acetabulum than in untreated cases, and it is often impossible to assess the prognosis in such cases. The results of surgery in failed infantile CDH are not so good as in those previously untreated (see Fig. 7.13).

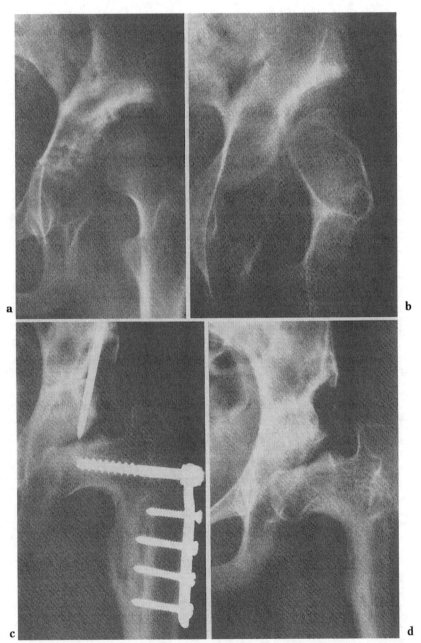

a

b

c

d

Fig. 7.13a–d. Failed juvenile CDH surgery, salvaged. **a** Juvenile CDH treated by Chiari osteotomy when 6 years old. Now 10 years. **b** Same patient 2 years later, further subluxation having developed at puberty. **c** Femoral shortening (2 cm) and varus osteotomy followed by pelvic osteotomy when 12 years old. **d** Two-year follow-up when 14 years old. The left hip has been stabilised in the original acetabulum. This means that hip replacement will be feasible later on, if the hip becomes stiff or painful.

Summary

Thus the treatment of juvenile hip displacement is surgical and must be courageous. There are four essential factors required for success:

1) There must be concentric reduction of the femoral head in an acetabulum at the level of the triradiate cartilage.

2) The blood supply to the proximal third of the femur must be preserved by retaining the integrity of the abductors and iliopsoas pedicle blood supplies.

3) The operative procedure must involve a decompression rather than a compression of the hip joint.

4) The acetabulum must be reorientated into its normal position.

References

Chiari K (1955) Ergebnisse mit der Beckenosteotomie als Pfannendachplastik. Orthop 87: 14

Colonna PC (1932) Congenital dislocation of the hip in older subjects. Based on a study of 66 open operations. J Bone Joint Surg 14: 277

Colonna PC (1953) Capsular arthroplasty for congenital dislocation of the hip. J Bone Joint Surg 35A: 179

Dega W, Krol J, Polakowski L (1959) Surgical treatment of congenital dislocation of the hip in children. J Bone Joint Surg 41A: 920

Eyre-Brook AL (1966) Treatment of congenital dislocation or subluxation of the hip in children over the age of 3 years. J Bone Joint Surg 48B(4): 682–692

Ganong W (1973) Review of medical physiology, 6th edn. Lange, U.S.A.

Glass A, Dunningham TH (1980) Capsular arthroplasty of the hip for congenital dislocation. Isr J Med Sci 16(4): 328

Hey Groves E (1928) The treatment of congenital dislocation of the hip. Robert Jones Birthday Volume, Oxford University Press, Oxford

Le Veuf J (1948) Results of open reduction on true congenital luxation of the hip. J Bone Joint Surg 30A: 875

Lloyd-Roberts GC (1978) quoted by Glass and Dunningham (1980) Capsular arthroplasty of the hip for congenital dislocation. Isr J Med Sci 16(4): 328

McFarland B (1956) Some observations on congenital dislocation of the hip. J Bone Joint Surg 38B(1): 54

Mitchell GP (1963) Arthrography in congenital displacement of the hip. J Bone Joint Surg 45B(1): 88–95

Mitchell GP (1970) Congenital dislocation of the hip. Scott Med J 15: 468

Pemberton PA (1965) Pericapsular osteotomy of the ilium for treatment of congenital subluxation and dislocation of the hip. J Bone Joint Surg 47A: 65–86

Pipino F (1980) Reduction, capsuloplasty and pelvic osteotomy in surgical treatment of inveterate congenital hip dislocation. Isr J Med Sci 16(4): 323

Perkins G (1928) Signs by which to diagnose congenital dislocation of the hip. Lancet 1: 648–650

Platt H (1953) Congenital dislocation of the hip. J Bone Joint Surg Editorial 35B: 339

Putti V (1933) Early treatment of congenital dislocation of the hip. J Bone Joint Surg 15: 16–21

Salter RB (1961) Innominate osteotomy in the treatment of congenital dislocation and subluxation of the hip. J Bone Joint Surg 43B: 518

Scaglietti O, Calandriello B (1962) Open reduction of congenital dislocation of the hip. J Bone Joint Surg 44B: 257

Steele HH (1977) Triple osteotomy of the innominate bone. Clin Orthop 122: 116–127

Tanner JM (1973) Textbook of paediatrics, 1st edn, pp 224–291. Churchill Livingstone, Edinburgh

Tanner JM, Whitehouse RH, Takaishi M (1966) Standards from birth to maturity for height, weight, height velocity and weight velocity in British children, Part 1. Arch Dis Child 41: 454

Tonnis D, Behrens K, Tscharini F (1981) A modified technique of the triple pelvic osteotomy: Early results. J Paediatr Orthop 1: 241–249

Trevor D (1957) Treatment of congenital dislocation of the hip. Editorial. J Bone Joint Surg 39B(4): 611

Trevor D (1960) Treatment of congenital hip dysplasia in older children. Proc R Soc Med (Section of Orthopaedics) 53: 481–490

Westin GW, Dallas TG, Watanabe BM, Ilfeld FW (1980) Skeletal traction vs. femoral shortening in treatment of older children with congenital hip dislocation. Isr J Med Sci 16(4): 318

8 Adult Congenital Acetabular Dysplasia with Subluxation of the Hip Joint

Some children have been born with their thighs luxated and have remained cripples. I shall not enter upon a discussion of those different causes. I shall only advise you wherever the dislocation is observed immediately to have recourse to the hand of the surgeon, for if this is neglected a callus will be formed in the dislocated part which will render the cure absolutely impossible.

Orthopaedia, Nicholas Andry (1743)

Although these words were written in the first orthopaedic textbook, even today they still hold true, despite the advances that have occurred in medical practice. This chapter is set aside in order to confirm Andry's original observation and also to relate our experience in the management of these most difficult adult patients.

There is no shortage of such candidates demanding treatment in our population. One in three or four of our long series have been treated for CDH during infant life, but their persistent dysplasia and subluxation is often a reflection of the failure of conservative treatment (see Fig. 8.1). The majority of patients, however, have no previous history of hip problems and their onset of symptoms is the first indication of congenital dysplasia of their hip joints.

In adult patients, a shallowness of the acetabulum can cause persistent discomfort and disablement in two ways. It affects the younger group of patients by producing an instability of the hip joint, due to an associated incarcerated limbus, or rarely when combined with a severe familial joint laxity. The instability produces muscle fatigue, which causes wasting and further muscle weakness. In older patients a persistent instability causes pain, which restricts activity and this can lead to an increase of body weight which in itself will aggravate the hip condition. This vicious circle leads to secondary osteoarthrosis.

Thus the two groups present in different ways.

Young Adults (15–25 Years)

Initially the symptoms are brought on by excessive physical activity, e.g. competitive sports and dancing. The pain is relieved by withdrawing from such pastimes, but the symptoms eventually affect everyday life. Yet rest pain is minimal, thus indicating a mechanical cause for their symptoms.

In many cases it is not unusual for the pain to be referred to the anteromedial aspect of the knee joint, adding to the mystery of the diagnostic problems in the adolescent female. These young women can also complain of locking or giving way of the affected leg due to a torn or incarcerated limbus in their dysplastic hip joint. Thus they represent a great risk, for the unwary surgeon will diagnose recurrent subluxation of the patella or even a tear of the medial meniscus. Some of our patients have been subjected to arthrograms and arthroscopy of the knee, and a few have had surgery, including a release incision of the vastus lateralis tendon of insertion into their patella, or sometimes a medial meniscectomy, with no alleviation of their symptoms. All the time a true diagnosis might have been made if the examiner had recognised a limitation of medial rotation of the affected leg, as compared to the opposite side. When the patient is lying prone it is easy to detect the "wasting of the buttock sign", especially in unilateral cases.

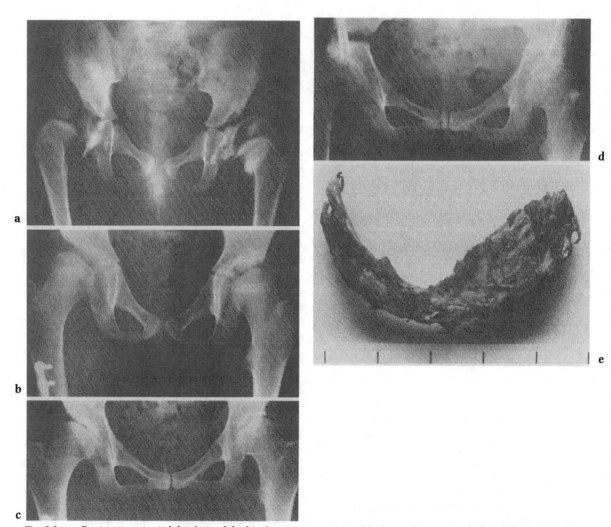

Fig. 8.1a–e. Persistent congenital dysplasia of the hip due to an incarcerated limbus. a Twenty-month-old girl in 1946. Bilateral hip displacement. Arthrogram of left hip reveals eccentric reduction due to an incarcerated limbus. b Six-year follow-up. Left hip has been treated conservatively and was thought to have stabilised with minimal persistent acetabular dysplasia. Right hip had a femoral osteotomy performed. c The same patient in 1979, 33 years after commencement of treatment. At this time the woman was crippled with pain in both hips, her symptoms being worse on the left than the right. d Bilateral pelvic osteotomies were performed to relieve her pain. On both sides an incarcerated and torn limbus was found at the time of arthrotomy and excised in order to improve the degree of containment of the femoral head. The limbus (e) was 5 cm in length.

There is much to be said for X-raying the pelvis and both hips of any young adult who complains of persistent discomfort in one or both knees, especially when there is no clinical evidence of internal derangement of the knee joint. In women there is a high chance of their pain being referred from the hip joint.

Later these young adults become crippled to such a degree that it is necessary for them to use crutches to help them get around and they become aware of acute discomfort in their groins on the affected side.

Older Age Group (35–45 Years)

Often these patients first experienced discomfort localised to their groins and later they refer to their buttock and thigh. Retrospectively some of the women have experienced a similar discomfort during previous pregnancies, but X-rays were not taken because of the foetus, and following delivery their pain disappeared spontaneously. Thus a sporadic type of pain is not unusual, but the symptoms eventually become more progressive. They begin to complain of pain at night time and during the day the discomfort interferes with walking and limits physical activities. Typically it is worse when they climb stairs or walk up inclined planes. They soon reach a point where they are forced to rest from everyday activities and may eventually have to use a stick or crutches to help them get around (see Fig. 8.2).

Clinical Signs

Most of these patients walk with a slight limp or a waddle and the Trendelenburg test is positive even if delayed until standing on the affected leg for a few minutes. The tendency for a dipping gait can be aggravated by apparent shortening due to flexion and adduction contractures of the affected hip joint in older patients.

There is usually evidence of wasting of the buttock muscles and sometimes the thigh, but this is often difficult to detect in bilateral cases. In unilateral hip dysplasia the flattening can be appreciated more by palpation with the flat of the hand, proving that such wasting can be felt before it is seen. The distance between the tip of the greater trochanter and anterior superior iliac spine may be diminished, even in cases of minimal subluxation. Leg length discrepancy is often present, but it is rarely more than 2 cm. The stigmata of familial joint laxity may be detected in half the women, but the prevalence is higher in men.

Limitation of movements in the affected hip is present in most cases. The restriction affects flexion, abduction, and medial rotation in this priority order. If the total range of movements is measured, the normal is 300°–340° in most adults, but in patients with painful congenital dysplasia of the hip the average is about 200°–250°.

Radiological Features

Evidence of congenital dysplasia and subluxation can usually be assessed more easily by observing the degree of exposure of the femoral head and the widening of the medial joint space in preference to measurement, even before Shenton's line is broken (see Fig. 8.1b). The average centre-edge angle of Wiberg is 13°, ranging from 0° to 17°, these readings being well below the 20° considered to be the lower level of normal range.

In the older age group, degenerative changes affect mainly the weight-bearing area, there being a loss of joint space sometimes associated with cysts in the acetabular roof and also in the femoral head (see Fig. 8.2a). There may be early osteophyte formation along the lateral margin of the acetabulum

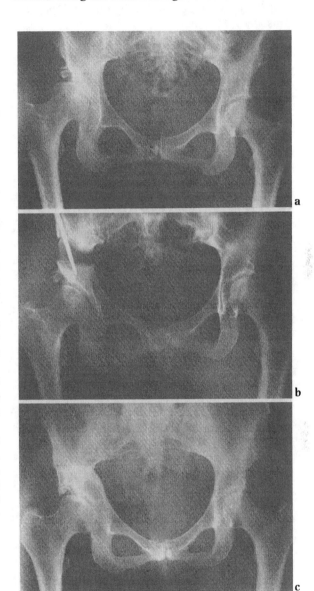

Fig. 8.2a–c. These are the X-rays of a 35-year-old woman in 1967 with crippling pain in her right hip. There was no previous history of hip disease. a X-rays revealed a congenital dysplasia and subluxation of her right hip with cystic degeneration of the femoral head. b A pelvic osteotomy was performed, but no arthrotomy was undertaken. c Six years later her right hip remained pain-free and she has regained almost a full range of movement. Note that Shenton's line has been restored, indicating complete stability of the hip and the cysts in the femoral head are becoming smaller in size. Subsequently she has remained pain-free to date and was last seen in 1982, 15 years from the time of pelvic osteotomy. There was no evidence of recurrence of her symptoms or signs.

and later arising from the inferior border of the articular surface of the femoral head (the cephalic osteophyte) and centrally around the fovea of the acetabulum. The latter tend to extrude the femoral head out of the socket and so increase the degree of instability and pain.

Management

The only conservative treatment successful in the relief of such crippling pain caused by congenital dysplasia and subluxation includes a combination of rest, partial weight-bearing on crutches and non-weight-bearing exercises either on a static exercise bicycle or by daily swimming. Excess weight is often a very important aggravating factor and a controlled loss provides a more lasting relief of discomfort. Yet such management affords only a temporary arrest, as the condition is "relentless in its final crippling results" (Hey Groves 1928).

Orthodox Surgical Alternatives

In adults with moderately severe degrees of osteoarthrosis secondary to a congenital hip dysplasia, with subluxation of the femoral head into a false acetabulum, various forms of femoral osteotomy have previously been advocated.

Lorenz (1919) was one of the first to suggest a subtrochanteric bifurcation osteotomy of the femur and this has already been described in Chap. 7, as performed by Ernest Hey Groves in 1928. Soon after, Alfred Schanz (1925) devised his valgus osteotomy at the same sub-trochanteric level, and his procedure has remained popular, as seen in Fig. 8.3. Later, Pauwels (1925) described his valgus femoral osteotomy (Pauwels II) performed at intertrochanteric level. His concept was to use the medial (cephalic) osteophyte on the femoral head as part of the articular weight-bearing surface. He believed this increased the articular congruity and decreased the stresses in the superolateral aspect of the acetabulum. Maquet developed this technique and in 150 cases he claimed 77% were good results with 83% pain-free hips, the effects lasting for at least 10 years (Langlais et al. 1979). These authors found that it was the hip joints in which the femoral heads were extruded by medial osteophytes that responded best to a Pauwels II osteotomy. Studying the postoperative X-rays of their patients and similar cases, the valgus osteotomy appears to stimulate the

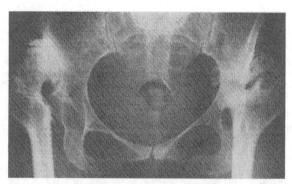

Fig. 8.3. X-ray of young adult, 25 years old. She had a bilateral Schanz femoral osteotomy performed when she was 8 years old. Both hips had remained relatively pain free despite a bilateral Trendelenburg gait. Total hip replacement will be difficult due to surgical deformation.

growth of the cephalic osteophyte, as if in order to occupy an increasing intra-articular space. Ronald Murray has described the development of the subarticular cartilaginous osteophyte as Nature's attempt to stabilise a weight-bearing joint or to prevent abnormal movements (personal communication). It could, therefore, be suggested that a valgus femoral osteotomy increased the stability of the hip, by first unstabilising the joint and thereby stimulating the development of a cephalic osteophyte with its stabilising effect.

Other surgical alternatives that are successful in relieving the crippling pain of a congenital dysplasia of the hip include Girdlestone's pseudo-arthroplasty (1943) involving excision of the femoral head and neck, plus the roof of the acetabulum, while an arthrodesis of the hip in unilateral CDH provides a permanent relief of pain. Such orthodox surgical measures provide a relief of discomfort at the expense of loss of either stability or movement. Pseudo-arthroplasty produces a very poor gait and arthrodesis rules out any successful future hip replacement. The temptation to proceed to early hip replacement, especially in the younger age group, is resisted by many surgeons because of the excess strain that these patients place upon their hips by youthful activities, and the subsequent high risk of revision replacement.

Adult Pelvic Osteotomy

In the present series, pelvic osteotomy has proved to be a very effective alternative in mature female and male patients (Wilkinson and Warr 1973). There is sufficient mobility of the pelvic articulations necessary to be able to displace the acetabulum to a degree that will stabilise the anterolateral subluxation of the hip joint. Excision of the limbus has also been found to be an important additional procedure, as it relieves the mechanical derangement of an incarcerated limbus in younger patients. The cosmetic and functional gain is superior to the orthodox methods mentioned above. There can be little doubt that pelvic osteotomy, performed by capable hands, is the surgical treatment of choice in carefully selected patients.

As experience in the surgical management of infants and juvenile patients with CDH increased, the challenge to apply the same principles to mature adults became formidable, the one fundamental change in the approach being that such major surgery can only be advised in adult patients who are crippled with pain. Adult pelvic osteotomy is never offered as a prophylactic procedure in patients with symptoms of merely nuisance value. This is unlike the previous policy outlined for infant and juvenile patients in which one is prepared to operate for prophylactic reasons even in the absence of pain.

Operative Technique. The same procedure is used as in infants, there being a few variations in the technique. Initially, a psoas release is performed through an adductor approach, as demonstrated in Fig. 8.4. This is because there is usually a contracture of the muscle in these age groups which is likely to aggravate any compression of the femoral head produced by the bony procedure. At the same time one can release any adductor contracture. There has been no residual disability arising from medial psoas release, but there are many benefits, including the absence of postoperative stiffness.

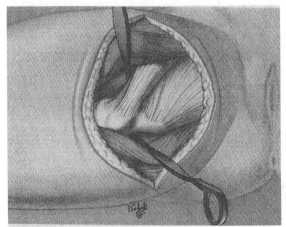

Fig. 8.4. Medial psoas release. Medial approach through adductor muscles to reveal lesser trochanter, allowing direct visual division of psoas tendon.

As there is no iliac apophysis in these age groups, the stripping of the iliac crest is more tedious and has to be performed methodically with diathermy and gentle elevation of the periosteum. Then the upper third of the iliac crest is excised, as in young children, to be used to fashion a smaller triangular graft which is inserted at the osteotomy site. This means there is a decrease in the overall height of the iliac crest, producing a comparative lengthening of the abductors and iliopsoas muscles.

In the young adults without any radiological evidence of osteoarthrosis, the hip joint is explored before osteotomy and it is usual to find a thickened and torn incarcerated limbus, as shown in Fig. 8.1d. As the limbus is thought to be a source of pain and recurrent derangement of the hip joint, it is excised with the aid of a Smillie's meniscectomy knife. This also increases the intra-articular space, facilitating the containment of the femoral head following the displacement of the acetabulum. Absorbable sutures are then placed in the capsule, but they are not tied until after the osteotomy has been performed.

The osteotomy is placed 1 cm above the capsular attachment of the hip joint, the bone being divided by a Gigli saw. It is then possible to flex the hip and knee and to put traction on the leg in order to displace the acetabulum forward and laterally. The defect created at the site of osteotomy is filled with a triangular bone graft, fashioned from the upper third of the iliac crest. Two stout stainless steel pins are inserted (O.E.E. Orthopaedics Limited, 1982). These stainless steel pins are coarsely threaded distally, so that their insertion compresses the osteotomy site. The thread also prevents postoperative extrusion of the pin.

Suction drains are placed inside and outside the pelvis to prevent any haematoma formation, which tends to delay healing of the wound with the secondary threat of wound sepsis. The drains are maintained for the first five postoperative days and then withdrawn. When the hip joint has been explored at the time of osteotomy, it is necessary postoperatively to place the patient in a one-and-a-half plaster hip spica for 6–8 weeks. This is in order to promote healing of the capsular incision and so prevent postoperative subluxation. In older patients with degenerative arthrosis, an arthrotomy is not performed and this means that there is no need for a plaster spica postoperatively, as the hip joint remains stable.

Partial weight-bearing is allowed on crutches after the plaster spica has been removed, but full weight-bearing is delayed until 12 weeks from surgery. If a bilateral osteotomy is being performed, an interval of 12 weeks is planned between the two sides. The pins are usually removed a year after surgery, but this is a minor out-patient operative procedure.

Outcome of Treatment

The initial overall success is similar in all patients, as the majority lose their pain immediately; yet there is a variation in the length of persistent pain relief in the two groups.

Young Adult Group. The results of pelvic osteotomy in these patients with no radiological evidence of degenerative arthrosis are excellent in the majority of cases. In 80% of patients the improvement is maintained. Painful locking and giving way of the hip joint, present in the majority of these patients, is nearly always relieved by arthrotomy and excision of the limbus and pelvic osteotomy. In the minority of patients, there was some late recurrence of discomfort, but this was never so severe as the pre-operative symptoms.

Donald Ainscow (personal communication 1983) reported a retrospective study of my patients. He compared the pre- and postoperative radiological assessments in a series of 30 patients, six having bilateral procedures. He found that 65% of hips had disruption of Shenton's line pre-operatively, but this was completely restored in two thirds of hips, with a subsequent permanent loss of symptoms. In the remaining third of patients, in which Shenton's line was only partially restored, there was a late recurrence of discomfort (see Fig. 8.5). The average centre-edge angle of Wiberg was 13° pre-operatively, but was increased to 25° post-operatively. Of nine patients with a final centre-edge angle of less than 20°, four had a recurrence of their pain. This outcome indicates that it is necessary to stabilise the joint and improve the acetabular cover by pelvic osteotomy, in order to obtain a complete and permanent loss of pain in this group of young patients.

Thus minor degrees of subluxation can be stabilised by lowering the femoral head to its normal level by relative lengthening of the abductors and flexors in the technique of pelvic osteotomy. This also allows a rotation of the acetabulum, laterally and forward, which prevents residual anterolateral subluxation.

The one radiological contra-indication to this form of pelvic osteotomy is subluxation of the femoral head, when the latter appears to be contained in a false acetabulum above the site of the original socket. Then a pelvic osteotomy with lateral displacement of the acetabulum is usually unsuc-

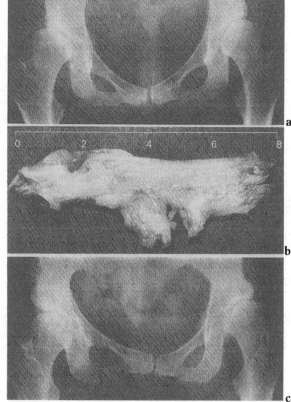

Fig. 8.5a–c. Persistent bilateral hip dysplasia and subluxation in 18-year-old woman who had been treated for bilateral CDH conservatively when she was 2 years old. **a** X-ray reveals bilateral hip dysplasia with poor covering of the femoral head and a break in Shenton's line on both sides. Early degenerative changes are developing in the left hip. **b** Bilateral pelvic osteotomies were performed and at the same time each hip joint was explored. A thickened inverted and torn limbus was found on each side. **c** The same patient 12 years later, having had two children since surgery. Both hips remained pain-free and she has a full range of movements on both sides. The right Trendelenburg test is negative, but the left is slightly positive. Note that anatomical concentric reduction has been attained on the right side with restoration of Shenton's line and full acetabular cover. On the left side the head has been stabilised in a false acetabulum with residual subluxation. The femoral head is not fully covered and Shenton's line remains broken. The persistent residual instability will lead to early degenerative changes, as concentric reduction was not attained at the time of surgery. In retrospect the pelvic osteotomy has aggravated the degree of residual subluxation.

cessful, as the subluxed femoral head is displaced more laterally and this does not correct the instability (see Fig. 8.5). To date, we have elected to perform a Chiari osteotomy (1970) in such patients and this has been followed by a surprising degree of remodelling, to produce an excellent socket. Unlike the juvenile patients, there has been no evidence of any progressive subluxation post-operatively, as skeletal maturity has been attained pre-operatively. Unfortunately, our patients have been left with a permanent limp and retrospectively this is thought to be due to a central displacement of the hip joint. The limp has not worried patients to any degree, as all are relieved of their discomfort and are very grateful for this.

Perhaps a femoral osteotomy, performed with a view to shortening the shaft of the femur, might be

a wise step before performing a pelvic osteotomy. Thus the femoral neck can be reduced to the level of the lower border of the superior pubic ramus, restoring Shenton's line, and any excess degree of femoral torsion can be corrected at the same time. Then one is able to rotate the acetabulum laterally over the femoral head and this might prove to be a more stabilising procedure for the subluxating hip joint. As in juveniles, the two osteotomies can be performed at the same time or the pelvic osteotomy may be delayed until 6 weeks after the femoral osteotomy.

Older Age Group. In the same series, there were 21 patients who first developed pain in their hips after the age of 35 years, and their X-rays at that time revealed acetabular dysplasia and signs of early osteoarthrosis. These older patients complained of rest pain, as well as discomfort aggravated by effort.

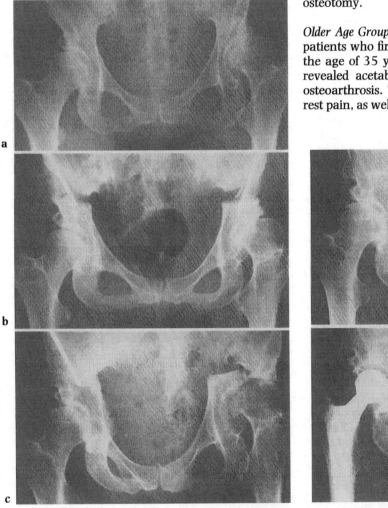

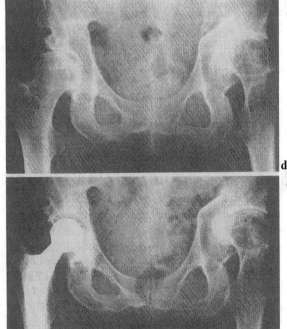

Fig. 8.6a–e. Persistent acetabular dysplasia and subluxation following conservative treatment of bilateral CDH in infant life. **a** Forty-year-old woman crippled with pain in both hips. Her right hip shows persistent dysplasia with minimal subluxation and slight loss of superior joint space. Her left hip reveals residual subluxation with cephalic osteophyte arising from the femoral head and also central osteophytes arising from the medial acetabular wall and causing the head to be extruded out of the acetabulum. There is a marked degree of loss of joint space over the summit of the femoral head. **b** A bilateral pelvic osteotomy was performed. Note that the right hip has reduced concentrically with restoration of Shenton's line and an apparent improvement in joint space. The left pelvic osteotomy has aggravated the degree of subluxation. **c** Two years later the right hip remains pain-free, but the left hip has become more painful and this has called for a Chiari osteotomy (aged 42 years). **d** Thirteen years later (age 55 years) her left hip remains pain-free despite positive Trendelenburg sign. Her right hip has become painful to a point where life is miserable and total range of movements have been reduced to 120°. **e** Total hip replacement performed on right side using a Muller straight-stemmed prosthesis. A large limbus was found incarcerated in the joint. There was no difficulty in performing the total replacement successfully.

Their symptoms were more than nuisance value and had begun to restrict their everyday activities. In five of the patients both hips were involved, sufficient to indicate pelvic osteotomy, giving a total of 26 treated hip joints. All but four of these patients had a complete relief of pain from surgery. This lasted on an average for 8 years, but the majority had a recurrence of discomfort after 10 years.

Radiologically the progress of degenerative changes was either arrested or slowed down and in some cases the improvement remained static for many years. There was radiological evidence of healing of bone cysts in both the acetabulum and femoral head, as seen in Fig. 8.2.

It was found that arthrotomy was not advantageous in this group, as half the patients developed a further loss of lateral joint space following the excision of the incarcerated limbus, as previously observed by Harris et al. (1979). Once again, in this group it was shown that the restoration of Shenton's line was an important factor with regard to prognosis, for when this was not accomplished progressive degenerative changes developed in spite of surgery, as seen in Fig. 8.6.

Half this older group came to total hip replacement within 10 years of pelvic osteotomy. No problem was experienced at the time of replacement. It was performed through an anterolateral approach in most cases and the previous pelvic osteotomy was found to produce a better amount of bone-stock, to provide sufficient support for the acetabular cup. It was unnecessary to use a free bone graft in order to stabilise the acetabular component (see Fig. 8.6).

In patients with a severe degree of acetabular dysplasia and secondary osteoarthrosis, in which the head was subluxated into a false acetabulum and had developed medial osteophytes, a Chiari osteotomy was preferred as pelvic osteotomy often increases the degree of instability. Although the Chiari procedure produced a relief of pain and secondary remodelling of the acetabulum and femoral head, these patients also developed a persistent limp, as described in the group of young adults (see Fig. 8.7).

Total Hip Replacement

Finally, there is a group of patients who do not present for treatment until they are more than 50 years old. Many have struggled throughout life with considerable disabilities in one or both hips. They are eventually forced to seek advice, because of increasing pain and crippledom, and are found to

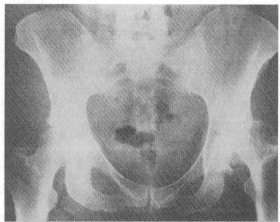

a

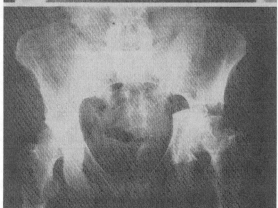

b

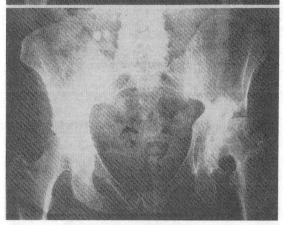

c

Fig. 8.7a–c. Congenital acetabular dysplasia of left hip, subluxation and moderately severe osteoarthritis. **a** X-ray of 42-year-old woman with severe pain in her left hip. Note the acetabular dysplasia with severe subluxation of the femoral head. There is a large cephalic osteophyte on the underpart of the femoral head and central osteophytes arising from the medial acetabular wall, causing an aggravation of the subluxation. **b** A Chiari osteotomy has been performed with central displacement of the acetabulum. **c** Eight-year follow-up. This patient's left hip has remained relatively pain free, but the Trendelenburg gait has persisted. Note the degree of remodelling and a persistent joint space. The inferior osteophytes appear to have increased in size and density.

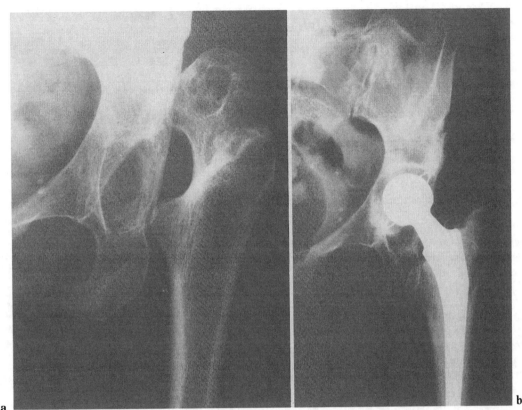

a   b

Fig. 8.8a,b. Persistent congenital dislocation of left hip in 55-year-old woman complaining of increasing pain over the past 2 years.
a Note the femoral head articulating with false acetabulum above the site of the original acetabulum. There is cystic degeneration
of the femoral head. **b** Salter approach with excision of the upper third of the iliac crest and relative lengthening of the flexors
and abductors, allowing the femoral head to be brought down to the level of the original acetabulum. This provided good bone
stock to cover the acetabular cup. Successful total hip replacement attained using a straight-stemmed Muller prosthesis.

have varying degrees of hip displacement with
secondary degenerative changes, as seen in Fig. 8.8.

In these cases it is essential to lower the femoral
head to the site of the primary acetabulum, in order
to be able to place the acetabular cup at a level
where there is sufficient bone-stock to support the
acetabular component, as well as to attain a normal
biomechanical relationship between the acetabular
and femoral components of the arthroplasty. This
lowering of the femoral head is attained by stripping
the flexors and abductor muscles from the inner and
outer aspects of the iliac bone, respectively, using
the Salter approach. Then the upper third of the iliac
crest is excised, to produce a relative lengthening
of the two muscle groups, in order to be able to bring
the femoral head and its prosthetic replacement
down to the appropriate level of the primary
acetabulum. Once again the restoration of Shenton's line produces the normal biomechanics, which
ensures a good future for the arthroplasty.

Summary

Thus in the major surgical reconstruction of the dysplastic and subluxated adult hip joint, we are not
faced with the two old enemies of surgical shock and
sepsis, and the risk to future bone growth does not
hang as a sword of Damocles over our heads. Also
the risk of postoperative infection and scar formation can be reduced and even eradicated by prefer-
ing bony correction to soft tissue release. Yet it is
still necessary to acknowledge the persistent
dangers of surgical tension and compression, if the
results of treatment are not to be prejudiced by stiffness and "precocious senility" of the joint.

The two diverse approaches to the surgical correction of congenital hip dysplasia and early secondary osteoarthrosis involve either the anatomical
restoration of joint stability or the functional
restoration of joint congruity.

Pauwels and Maquet opted for the functional restoration by performing a valgus osteotomy at the expense of stability. As a consequence this stimulated a natural growth of osteophytes, resulting in further stability.

The proposed alternative method of reconstruction involves the lowering of the femoral head to the level of the primary acetabulum, using the various surgical techniques described for juvenile cases in Chap. 7. Following the restoration of Shenton's line, the hip can be stabilised by pelvic osteotomy, which allows the rotation of the acetabular roof laterally and forward without encroaching on or compressing the articular surfaces.

Residual instability after major surgical reconstruction causes muscle contraction and stiffness, restricting the joint movement which is essential for physiological recovery. If this threat to articular recovery is removed, residual bony incongruity of the articular surfaces recedes owing to the remarkable remodelling potential possessed by living bone. As stability of a weight-bearing joint is ensured by concentricity of reduction, it is rewarded by a good return of function, which in turn is followed by remodelling of the articular components.

Even if the outcomes of these two diverse approaches are equally successful within the first 10 years, the anatomical correction of hip deformation holds out a better prospect for successful total hip replacement in later years, if this ever becomes a necessity.

References

Andry N (1973) Orthopaedia. Facsimile reproduction of the first edition in English, London 1743. Lippincott, Philadelphia and Montreal

Chiari K (1970) Pelvis osteotomy for hip subluxation. J Bone Joint Surg 52B: 174

Girdlestone GR (1943) Acute pyogenic arthritis of the hip: Operation giving free access and effective drainage. Lancet 1: 419

Harris W, Bourne R, Indong A (1979) Intra-articular acetabular labrum: a possible etiological factor in certain cases of osteoarthritis of the hip. J Bone Joint Surg 61A(4): 510

Hey Groves E (1928) The treatment of congenital dislocation of the hip. Robert Jones Birthday Volume, Oxford University Press, Oxford

Langlais F, Roure J-L, Maquet P (1979) Valgus osteotomy in severe osteoarthritis of the hip. J Bone Joint Surg 61B(4): 424

Lorenz A (1919) Über die Behandlung der irrepossiblen angeborenen Hüftluxationen und der Schenkelhalspseudo arthrosen mittels Gabelung (Bifurkation des oberen Femurendes). Wien Klin Wochenschr 32: 997

Pauwels F (1925) Der Schenkelhalsbruch, ein mechanisches Problem. Enke, Stuttgart

Schanz A (1925) Über die nach Schenkelhalsbruchen zurückbleibenden Gestveringen. Dtsch Med Wochenschr 51: 730–732

Wilkinson JA, Warr A (1973) Pelvic osteotomy for osteoarthritis of the hip joint. Proc R Soc Med 66(3): 241–242

Subject Index